Atlas of
CT Pathology

Atlas of
CT Pathology

Deborah L. Durham, BS, RT(R) (MR) (CT)
Forsyth Technical Community College
Winston-Salem, North Carolina

W.B. SAUNDERS COMPANY
A Division of Harcourt Brace & Company
Philadelphia ■ London ■ Toronto ■ Montreal ■ Sydney ■ Tokyo

W.B. SAUNDERS COMPANY
A Division of Harcourt Brace & Company

The Curtis Center
Independence Square West
Philadelphia, Pennsylvania 19106

Library of Congress Cataloging-in-Publication Data

Durham, Deborah L.
Atlas of CT pathology / Deborah L. Durham.

p.   cm.

ISBN 0–7216–6415–6

1. Tomography—Atlases.   I. Title.
   [DNLM: 1. Pathology—atlases.   2. Tomography, X-Ray Computed—
   atlases.   QZ 17 D961a 1997]

   RC78.7.T6D867 1997   616.07′572—dc20

DNLM/DLC   96–29334

ATLAS OF CT PATHOLOGY   ISBN 0–7216–6415–6

Printed in the United States of America.

Last digit is the print number: 9   8   7   6   5   4   3   2   1

To Barry Burns, Janice Keene, Robert Thorpe, and Gilbert Turner
Need I say more?

Preface

The most important goal of this atlas is to provide a coffee table book–like, fun approach for CT technologists and students to learn about the disease processes they are helping to diagnose. Images included are the "real" thing, not "doctored" as in so many other texts.

A brief overview of CT technology is given to help in understanding the pathologies seen using a variety of CT imaging techniques. Reference tables are in Chapter 1 to assist with review of the pathology charts for each disease process.

The atlas chapters were determined according to the specifications given by the American Registry of Radiologic Technologists for their national examination on computed tomography. This volume can thereby be used as a learning and teaching tool for this examination.

Acknowledgments

I wish to thank and acknowledge all those who were instrumental in the preparation of this atlas.

I am especially grateful to John Briggs for all of the photography of the scans. He did a tremendous job.

Thanks to Sherri Poore for helping with the computer and the word processing of the manuscript.

A special thanks to the CT technologists at Forsyth Memorial Hospital and North Carolina Baptist Hospital in Winston-Salem, North Carolina, for all their help. Thanks also to the CT technologists at Community General Hospital in Thomasville, North Carolina, and at Hawthorne Imaging Center in Winston-Salem, North Carolina.

Thanks to the CT technologists at High Point Regional Hospital in High Point, North Carolina—Cindy, Dwayne, Kathy, Marcine, and Sherry—for helping me gather CT images and for always looking for new examples of pathologies.

A special thanks to James Sanderford, MD, for being my medical advisor for this atlas and for giving me needed counsel.

I am very grateful to my present and previous students for all their questions. The students were the inspiration for this atlas—to help them learn more about the different disease processes. This volume, it is hoped, will benefit students in all of the health-related technologies.

I am most grateful to all my friends and fellow faculty members and to my dean for their encouragement and support for this project.

A simple thank you to Jim and Luli for all they have done for the past 18 years.

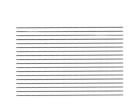

Contents

CHAPTER ONE

Reference Review

CT is becoming a more complicated technology with the advent of newer scan techniques. CT uses radiation (as in plain film radiography) to obtain axial (transverse) sections through the body. To understand how this is accomplished, a discussion of the equipment involved is needed.

The CT gantry with the patient couch is located in the actual procedure room. The CT gantry looks like a giant "doughnut" sitting on its side, with the patient couch operating from one side of it. The patient couch raises up and moves horizontally through the "doughnut hole" as x-ray slices are taken (Fig. 1–1). The couch is constructed of materials to allow x-ray transmissions without any interference. The mechanically stable x-ray tube and the detectors are located inside the covers of the gantry. The detectors act as the "film" by measuring the attenuation (x-ray energy

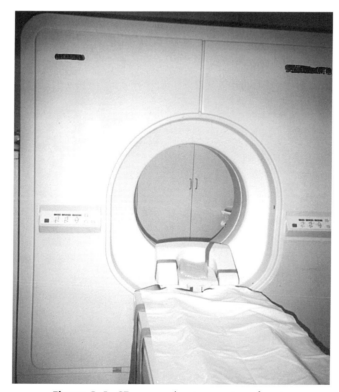

Figure 1–1. CT scanner showing aperture of gantry

that moves through the patient) properties of the tissues. The x-ray tube and detector array are mechanically coupled in third-generation scanners. They rotate 360 degrees around the patient, gathering data for a slice. The x-ray beam is pulsed on and off during this rotation. All of these operations are controlled at the computer console (Fig. 1–2).

The attenuation information of the tissue is converted by the detectors to an electrical signal that can be channeled into the array processor computer for image calculation (Table 1–1). This electrical signal is changed into numerical form by the analog-to-digital converter in order for the computer to "read" the information. Image reconstructions are calculated using algorithms or formulas of complex mathematical equations. Three major algorithms are used in CT: standard, bone, and detail. Each algorithm has different mathematic equations to reconstruct the images a certain way. To display a black, white, and gray image on the monitor, attenuation factors from the tissues in the slice are used to calculate CT numbers, which together create a gray scale for the slice. The CT number corresponds with a pixel in the image, which matches a voxel (volume of tissue) attenuation value. All attenuation values are based on that of water. Many pixels make up the image, representing many voxels. White areas represent high x-ray attenuation; black areas represent the opposite: low attenuation. Gray areas mean the tissue is somewhere in between high and low x-ray attenuation.

Procedure

A patient undergoing a CT scan is positioned on the patient couch. A scout, or "baby x-ray" film, is taken of the intended area. From this scout, the axial slices can be plotted according to the proper protocol for the disease process (Table 1–2). The table

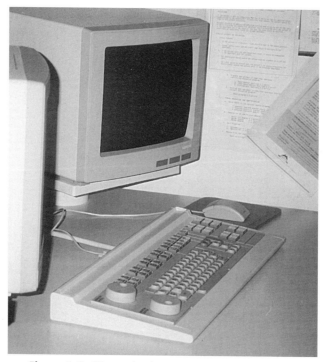

Figure 1–2. CT console where scan sequence is controlled

Table 1–1. **Parameter Chart**

Parameter	Description
Kilovolts (kVp)	One thousandth of force that will produce a current of 1 A in circuit with resistance of 1 Ω
Milliampere (mA)	One thousandth of an ampere
Milliampere-seconds (mAs)	The number of electrons applied to cathode of x-ray tube multiplied by exposure time in seconds; determines amount of x-ray energy produced
Scan field of view	Area scanned by machine
Display field of view	Area of scan field of view to be displayed on monitor
Matrix	Rows and columns of pixels (two dimensional) representing voxels (three-dimensional volume of tissue) in image
Slice thickness	The thickness of the slice
Slice gap	The distance between slices
Algorithm	Mathematical equations (formulas) used to reconstruct data a certain way Standard: used for brain, chest, abdomen, pelvis Detail: used for edge detail (e.g., for neck and face); window widths and window levels are moderate Bone: used for detail but not for contrast resolution (e.g., sinuses, temporal bones, extremity bones); window widths and window levels are widened
Window width	Range of gray scale as determined by the CT numbers representing the attenuations of the tissues: water, 0; air, −1000; bone, 1000
Window level	Center of gray scale

moves to the correct position and a slice is scanned; the table moves and another slice is scanned; and so on. When a patient undergoes a CT scan, an oral or an intravenous (IV) contrast, or a combination, is used.

Contrasts

Oral contrasts are used to line and highlight the gastrointestinal (GI) tract. They appear whitish on the scans and help differentiate abnormalities from normal bowel. Two kinds of oral contrasts are available: a water-soluble compound and a dilution of barium (1.5–3.0%). Barium used for upper GIs and in barium enemas is too concentrated and causes streaks on the CT image and thus degrades quality. The patient drinks the contrast well before the examination and then a cup immediately before the procedure. The normal total amount consumed is approximately 900 to 1000 mL.

Two types of IV contrasts are used for CT scanning: nonionic and ionic. Both contain iodine to highlight organs, vessels, and lesions. Nonionics are less irritating to the blood in the body; therefore, they cause fewer reactions. Nonionics are hypo-osmolaric, whereas ionics are hyperosmolaric (more active particles per solution). Most of the time, the IV contrast is injected through an angiocatheter in a vein by a pressure injector (Fig. 1–3). The pressure injector can be programmed to give a bolus of contrast at a specific time or to infuse a steady rate of contrast. The total amount of IV contrast given to an adult is about 100 to 150 mL.

Table 1–2. **Common Protocols**

Area	Protocol
Routine head (standard)	Lateral scout 4–5 mm slices through posterior fossa 7 mm throughout rest of head mAs = 340 kVp = 120 Matrix = 256 × 256 DFOV = 220 mm Usually done without and with IV contrast
Routine chest (standard)	Anterior to posterior scout/7 mm from top of apex of lungs down through the liver if questionable cancer mAs = 275 kVp = 130 Matrix = 256 × 256, 512 × 512 DFOV = 400 mm Usually with IV contrast
Routine abdomen-pelvis (standard)	Anterior to posterior scout/7 mm from top of diaphram down to the symphysis pubis mAs = 330 kVp = 120 Matrix = 256 × 256, 512 × 512 DFOV = 400 mm Usually with IV contrast Oral contrast

Sinus (bone)
Minisinus (one slice is done
  through each sinus area)
	Lateral scout
	4–5 mm from top of frontal sinus down through end of sphenoid
	  sinus
	mAs = 340
	kVp = 120
	Matrix = 256 × 256, 512 × 512
	DFOV = 150 mm
	IV contrast dependent

Facial bones (bone)	Lateral scout/anterior to posterior scout 3–4 mm through facial bones mAs = 340 kVp = 120 Matrix = 256 × 256, 512 × 512 DFOV = 150 mm IV contrast dependent
Spine (standard)	Lateral scout 3–4 mm angled through disc spaces mAs = 550 kVp = 120 Matrix = 256 × 256, 512 × 512 DFOV = 180 mm IV contrast dependent Spine usually done after myelography with contrast in thecal sac

mAs = milliampere-seconds; kVp = kilovolt (peak); DFOV = display field of view; IV = intravenous.

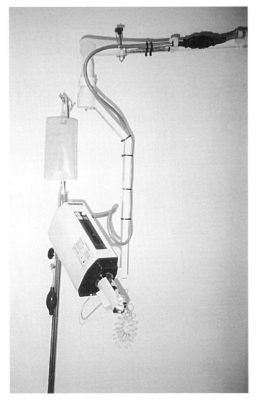

Figure 1–3. CT pressure injector for intravenous contrast

Spiral Computed Tomographic Scan

A reasonably new technique in CT that merits discussion is the spiral or helical or volumetric scanning technique. It allows a volume of data to be gathered with one breath hold by the patient. Spiral CT is defined as the continuous feed of the patient couch into the gantry with continuous rotation of the x-ray tube. The volume of data is acquired and can then be reconstructed using the different slice thicknesses needed. Most often it is used to scan the chest and abdomen, especially to look at the vessels in the chest and the liver.

Summary

With this brief introduction of how CT operates to produce transverse images from x-ray attenuations of the body tissues, this volume should provide a good learning tool for CT pathologies.

Bibliography

Applegate E. The sectional anatomy learning system. Philadelphia: WB Saunders, 1991.

Barrett C, Anderson L, Holder L. Primer of sectional anatomy with MRI and CT correlation. Baltimore, MD: Williams & Wilkins, 1994.

Barrett C, Poliakoff S, Holder L. Primer of sectional anatomy with MRI and CT correlation. Baltimore, MD: Williams & Wilkins, 1990.

Chandrasoma P, Taylor CR. Concise pathology, 2nd ed. Norwalk, CT: Appleton & Lange, 1995.

Firooznia H, Golimbu C, Rafil M. MRI and CT of the musculoskeletal system. St. Louis, MO: Mosby-Year Book, 1992.

Latchaw R. MR and CT imaging of the head, neck, and spine, 2nd ed. St. Louis, MO: Mosby-Year Book, 1991.

Lipman J. Quick reference to radiology. East Norwalk, CT: Appleton & Lange, 1995.

McDonough J, ed. Stedman's concise medical dictionary, 2nd ed. New York: Prentice Hall General Reference & Travel (Webster's New World), 1994.

Mulvihill ML. Human diseases—a systemic approach. Norwalk, CT: Appleton & Lange, 1955.

Robbins S, Cotran R, Kumar V. Pocket companion to Robbins pathologic basis of disease. Philadelphia: WB Saunders, 1991.

Seeram E. Computed tomography: physical principles, clinical applications and quality control. Philadelphia: WB Saunders, 1994.

CHAPTER TWO

Head and Neck

Chart 2–1. **Head and Neck** (Figs. 2–1, 2–2)

Pathology	Pituitary lesion
Description	Mass arising from either the anterior or the posterior lobe of pituitary gland; variation in size: microadenoma ($<$1 cm) or macroadenoma ($>$1 cm)
Symptoms	Blurred vision Increased prolactin levels
Suggested protocols	Routine head Thin slices through sella Coronal reconstructions
Appearance	Sella turcica area widened
Contrast	Gland enhances immediately after contrast; lesions do not; delay scan (30–40 minutes after contrast) shows lesions enhanced with the gland unenhanced

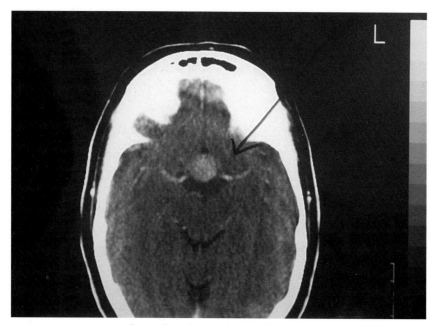

Figure 2–1. Pituitary lesion with contrast

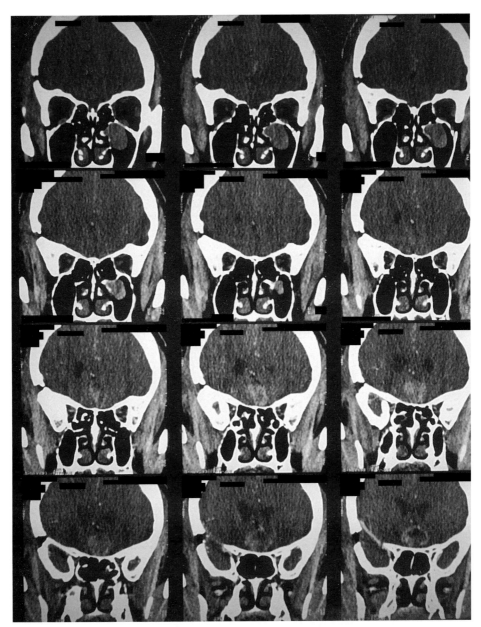

Figure 2-2. Pituitary lesion: reconstructed coronals with contrast

Chart 2–2. **Head and Neck** (Figs. 2–3 to 2–6)

Pathology	Hydrocephalus
Description	Increased abnormal volume of cerebrospinal fluid causing enlarged ventricles; occurs because of possible blockage in system resulting from congenital malformations, infections, subarachnoid hemorrhage, and other lesions
Symptoms	Dementia, gait disturbance, headache, nausea
Suggested protocols	Routine head
Appearance	Cerebrospinal fluid–filled ventricles are very large and black, displacing brain tissue
Contrast	To enhance a lesion possibly causing blockage

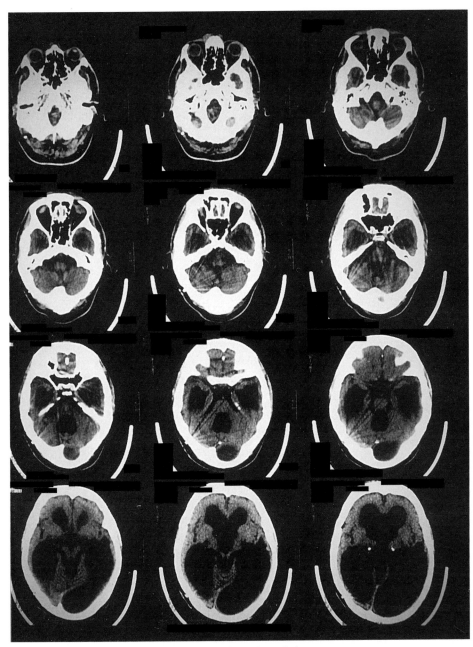

Figure 2–3. Hydrocephalus

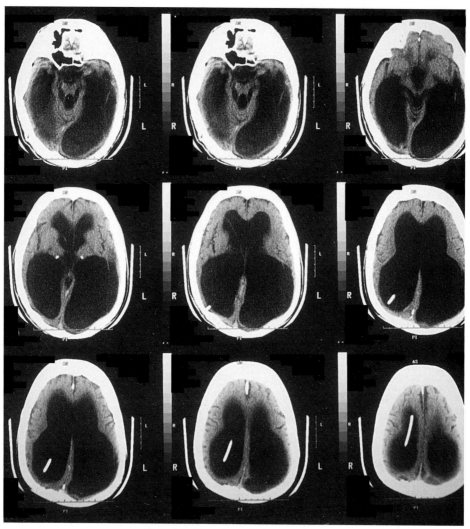

Figure 2–4. Hydrocephalus with shunt

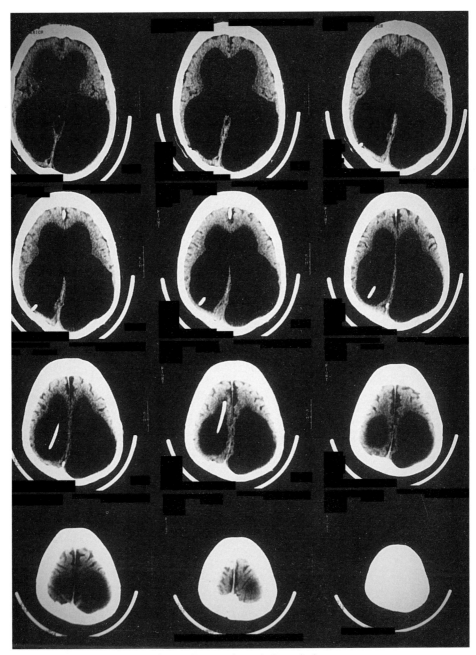

Figure 2–5. Hydrocephalus with shunt

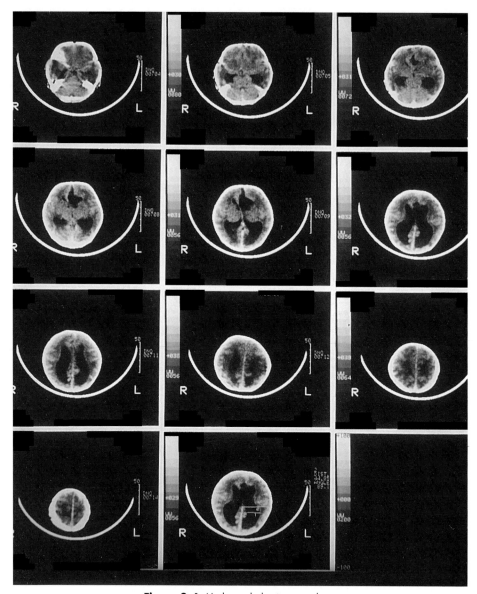

Figure 2–6. Hydrocephalus in a newborn

Chart 2–3. **Head and Neck** (Fig. 2–7)

Pathology	Pneumocephalus
Description	Air has gotten into brain tissue from a surgical process or from trauma
Symptoms	Pressure on brain tissue as a result of air compressing cerebral cortex
Suggested protocols	Routine head
Appearance	Air appears black into the gray brain tissue
Contrast	Dependent on radiologist

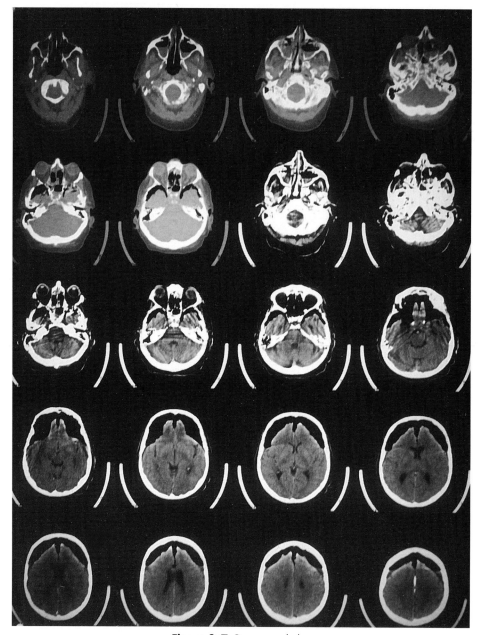

Figure 2–7. Pneumocephalus

Chart 2–4. **Head and Neck** (Figs. 2–8, 2–9)

Pathology	Cerebellar tissue changes
Description	Psychotropic drugs affect the central nervous system; chronic toxic effects on tissue
Symptoms	Seizures, personality changes, loss of consciousness
Suggested protocols	Routine head
Appearance	Attenuation changes in brain tissue as a result of chronic drug abuse and toxicity
Contrast	To differentiate from stroke or lesion

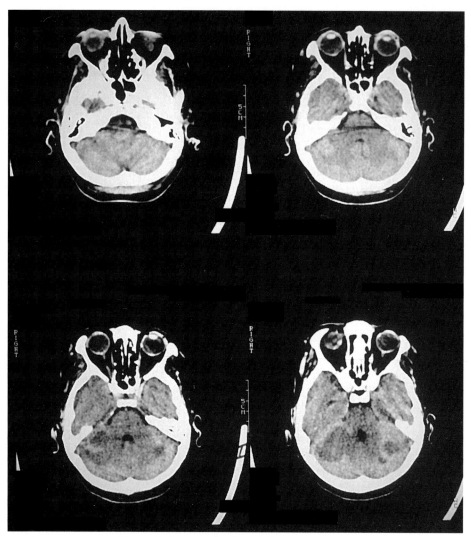

Figure 2–8. Drug-related cerebellar tissue changes

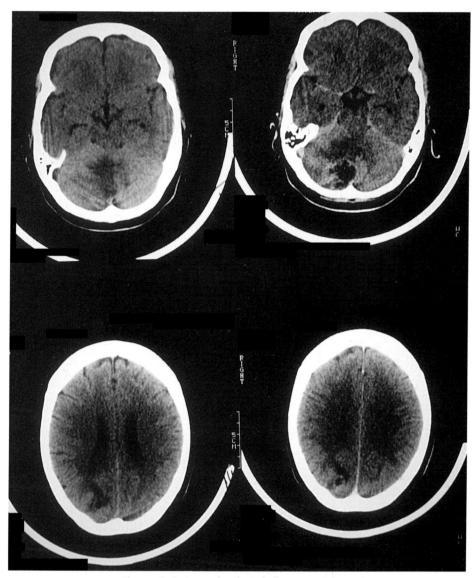

Figure 2–9. Drug-related cerebellar tissue changes

Chart 2–5. **Head and Neck** (Figs. 2–10, 2–11)

Pathology	Right parietal stroke Right occipital stroke
Description	Brain tissue becomes ischemic as a result of atherosclerotic disease, thrombus, embolus, or arterial spasm; tissue infarcts and is destroyed; edema surrounds the area and can cause some of the neurologic deficits
Symptoms	Sudden loss of neurologic function Right parietal stroke: contralateral hemiparesis, aphasia, usually associated with middle cerebral artery Right occipital stroke: visual loss, usually associated with posterior cerebral artery
Suggested protocols	Routine head
Appearance	Stroke does not visualize on CT scan during first 48 hours unless hemorrhagic stroke; attenuation changes from ischemia appear in about 3 days; CTs are performed immediately when symptoms appear to determine treatment
Contrast	Dependent on radiologist

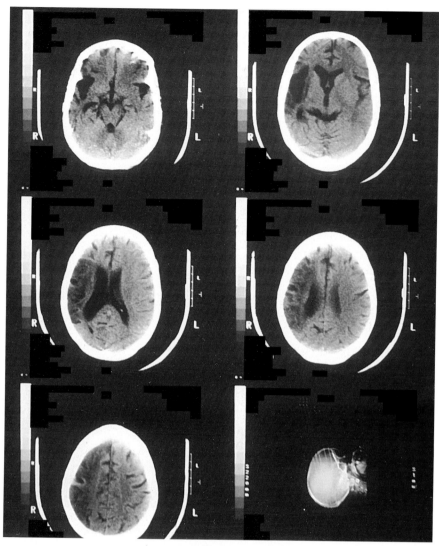

Figure 2-10. Right parietal stroke

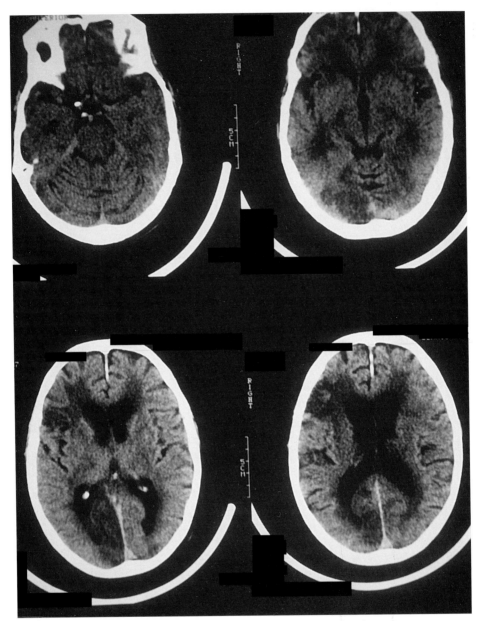

Figure 2-11. Right parietal stroke, right occipital stroke

Chart 2–6. **Head and Neck** (Fig. 2–12)

Pathology	Left versus right parietal stroke (new versus old)
Description	Strokes are caused by ischemia to the brain tissue from atherosclerotic disease, thrombus, embolus, or arterial spasm; brain tissue is destroyed and edema surrounds the area
Symptoms	Contralateral hemiparesis and aphasia
Suggested protocols	Routine head
Appearance	Old strokes appear almost black, and a newer stroke (2–3 weeks) is a darker gray but not black; this comes from different attenuations of the tissue dependent on age of stroke
Contrast	Dependent on radiologist

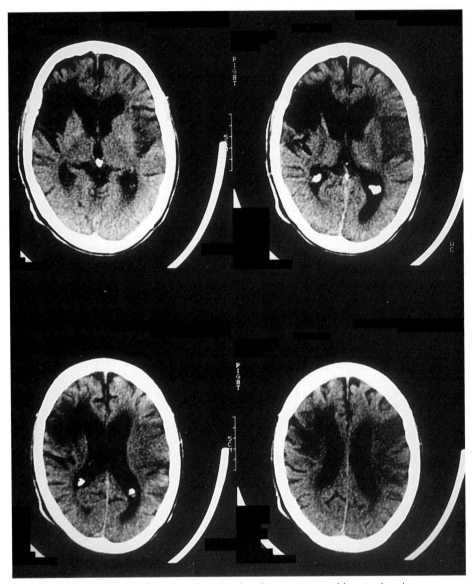

Figure 2–12. Left versus right parietal stroke, new versus old parietal stroke

Chart 2–7. **Head and Neck** (Fig. 2–13)

Pathology	Hemorrhagic stroke
Description	Site of bleeding usually from lenticulostriate arteries; increased pressure from atherosclerotic disease, thrombus, and embolus
Symptoms	Headache, contralateral neurologic deficits
Suggested protocols	Routine head
Appearance	Blood appears white and surrounding edema darker on head scans
Contrast	Dependent on radiologist

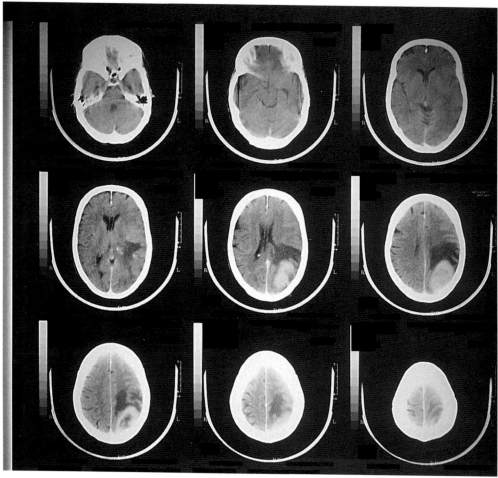

Figure 2–13. Hemorrhagic stroke

Chart 2–8. **Head and Neck** (Figs. 2–14 to 2–17)

Pathology	Subarachnoid hemorrhage
Description	Blood in space between arachnoid and pia mater, usually caused by rupture or leak of a berry aneurysm in the circle of Willis
Symptoms	Sudden onset of "bursting headache," vomiting, neck pain, and loss of consciousness
Suggested protocols	Routine head
Appearance	Blood appears white on head scans; scan resembles a "postcontrast" scan
Contrast	Dependent on radiologist

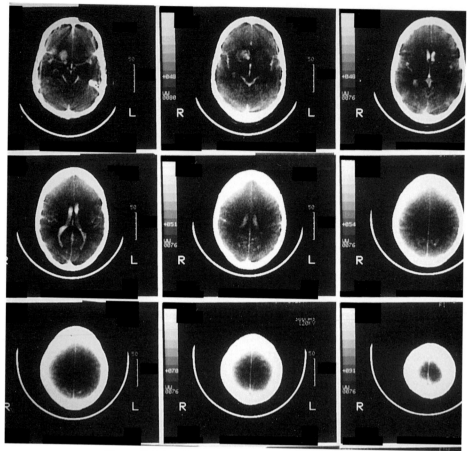

Figure 2–14. Subarachnoid hemorrhage with aneurysm

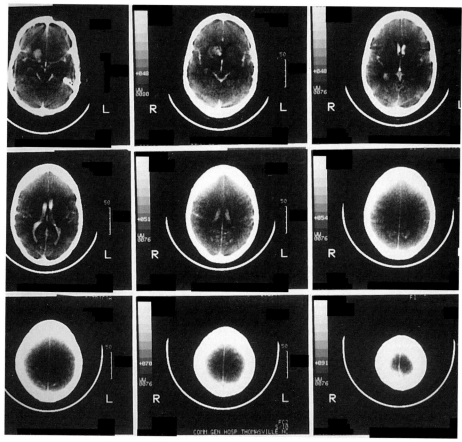

Figure 2–15. Subarachnoid hemorrhage with aneurysm

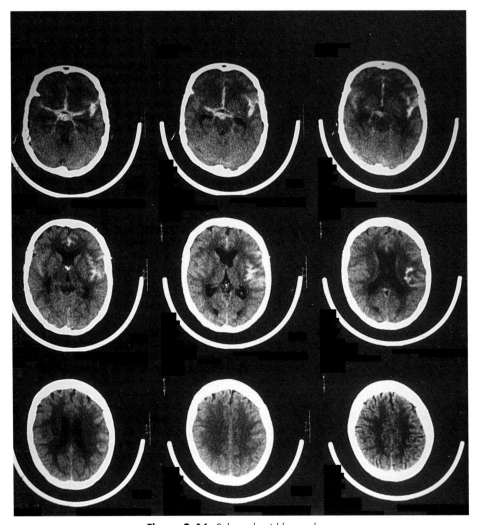

Figure 2-16. Subarachnoid hemorrhage

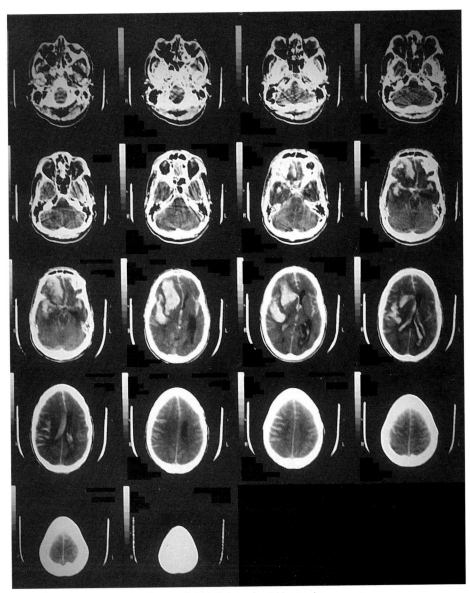

Figure 2-17. Subarachnoid hemorrhage

Chart 2–9. **Head and Neck** (Figs. 2–18 to 2–21)

Pathology	Intracerebral hemorrhage
Description	Secondary to hypertension occurring after age 40 years; most common site is around the basal ganglia (gray matter) and the internal capsule (white matter tract) because of rupture of lenticulostriate arteries
Symptoms	Abrupt onset of headache, trauma, neurologic deficits, with possible loss of consciousness
Suggested protocols	Routine head
Appearance	Blood appears white on head scan
Contrast	To differentiate bleed versus other lesions

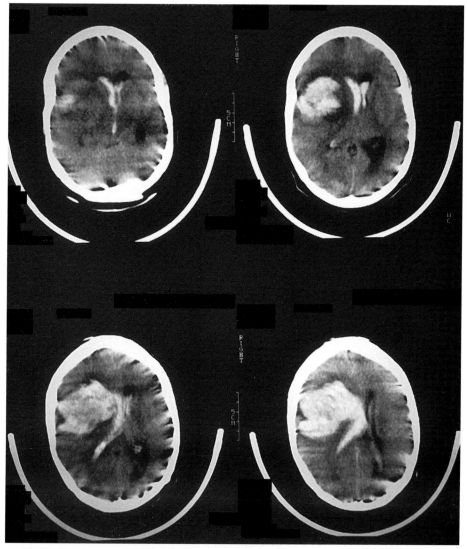

Figure 2-18. Intracerebral hemorrhage

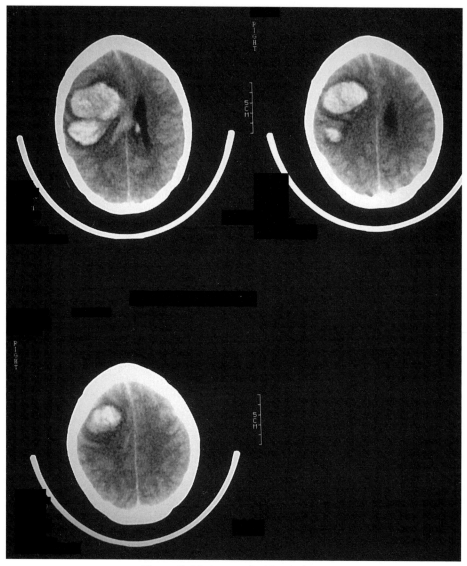

Figure 2–19. Intracerebral hemorrhage

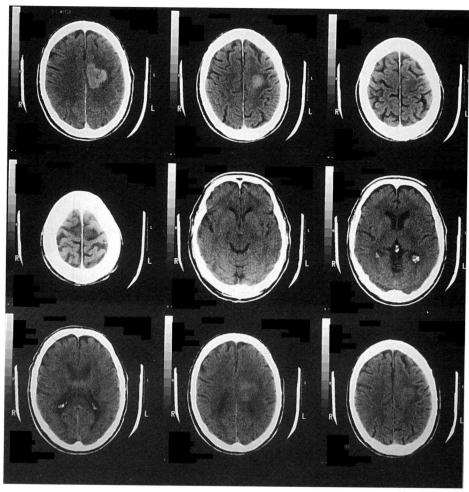

Figure 2–20. Intracerebral hemorrhage

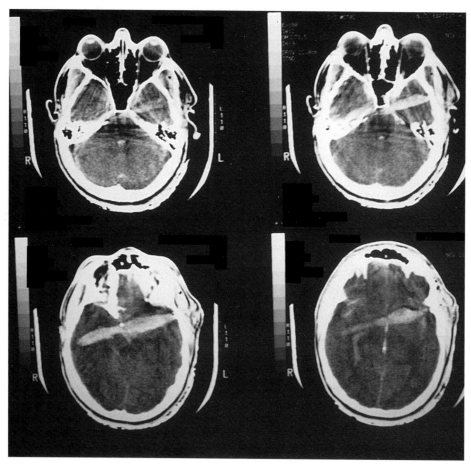

Figure 2-21. Intracerebral hemorrhage from knife wound

Chart 2–10. **Head and Neck** (Figs. 2–22, 2–23)

Pathology	Arteriovenous malformation (AVM) with skull defect
Description	Tangle of abnormal vessels with varying diameters that have large feeding arteries and large draining veins; occurs mostly in cerebral hemispheres
Symptoms	Headache, pulsing in ear
Suggested protocols	Routine head with thin slices through AVM
Appearance	Contrast appears white on head scan so tangle of vessels is visualized; pulsing of AVM has caused a dark skull defect next to AVM
Contrast	To visualize AVM

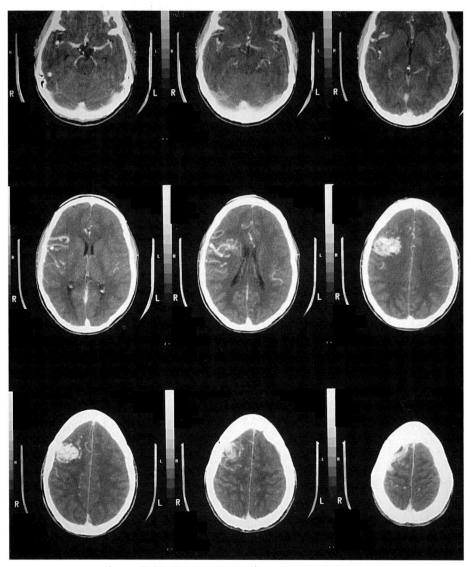

Figure 2–22. Arteriovenous malformation with skull defect

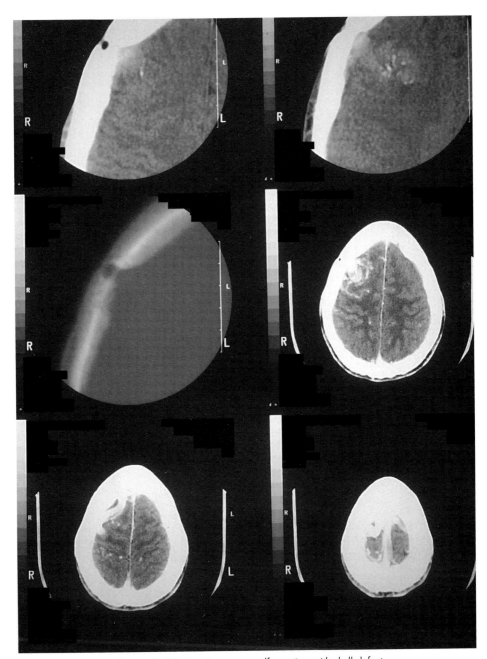

Figure 2-23. Arteriovenous malformation with skull defect

Chart 2–11. **Head and Neck** (Figs. 2–24 to 2–26)

Pathology	Severe trauma to head
Description	Severe crushing injury
Symptoms	Trauma
Suggested protocols	Routine head
Appearance	Temporoparietal portion of skull is pushed into brain tissue, with extensive bleeding (white) as a result of rupture of vessels
Contrast	Not necessary

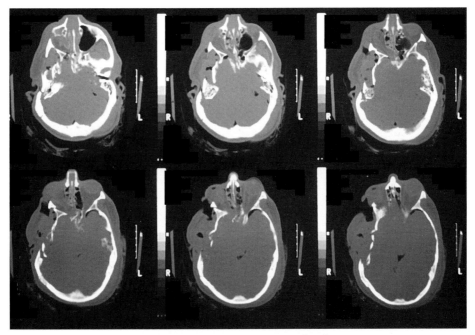

Figure 2-24. Severe trauma to head

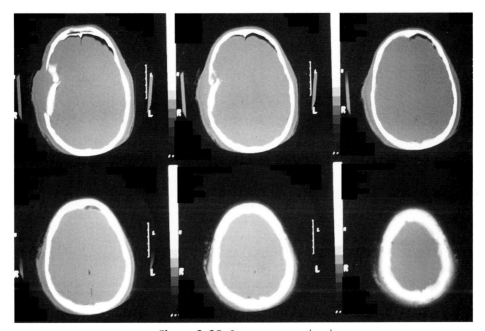

Figure 2-25. Severe trauma to head

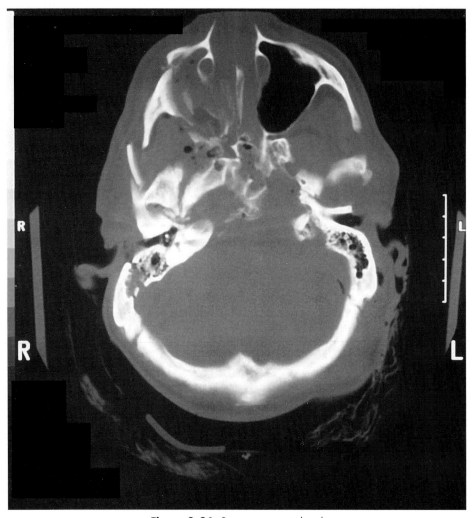

Figure 2–26. Severe trauma to head

Chart 2–12. **Head and Neck** (Figs. 2–27, 2–28)

Pathology	Cholesteatoma
Description	Squamous epithelium forms a pearly white mass from acute and chronic inflammation; usually occurs in middle ear
Symptoms	Imbalance, earache, dizziness
Suggested protocols	Routine brain Reconstructions with bone algorithm and filmed with wide window widths and levels
Appearance	Appears white in gray internal and middle ear area
Contrast	To enhance infectious process

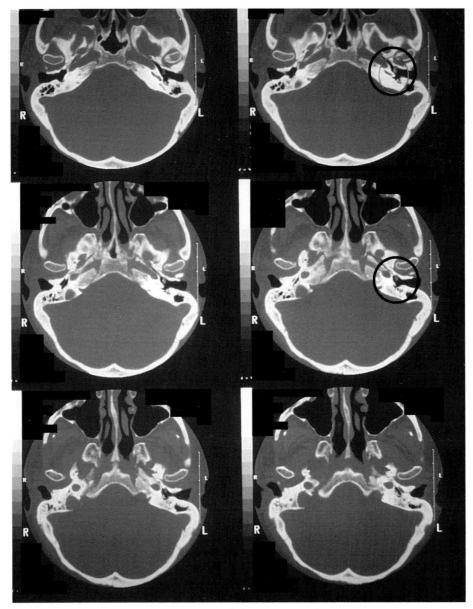

Figure 2–27. Cholesteatoma (axial)

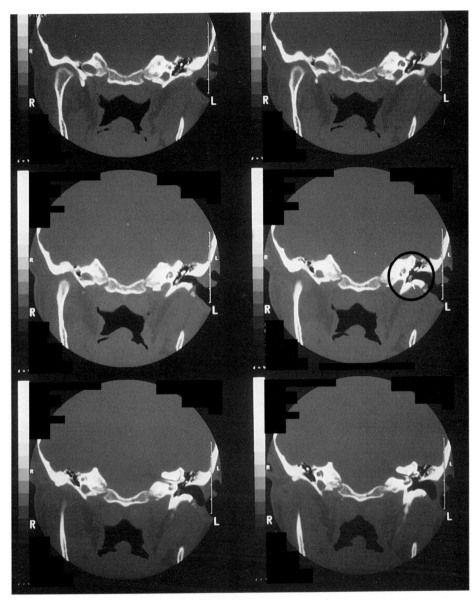

Figure 2–28. Cholesteatoma (coronal)

Chart 2–13. **Head and Neck** (Fig. 2–29)

Pathology	Maxillary sinus disease
Description	Inflammation of maxillary sinus, complication from acute rhinitis as a result of clogged nasal passages caused by nasal edema
Symptoms	Headache, fever, cervical lymph node enlargement
Suggested protocols	Routine sinus Minisinus
Appearance	Gray inflammatory process appears instead of normal black air in maxillary sinus
Contrast	Dependent on radiologist

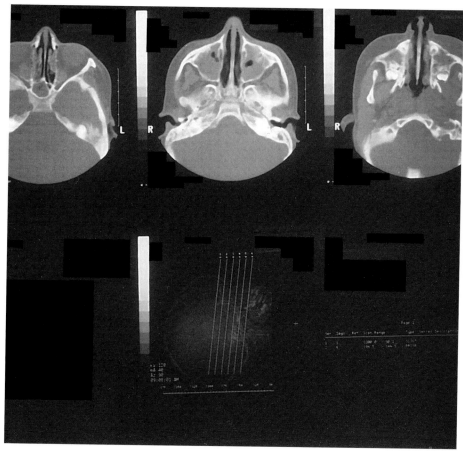

Figure 2-29. Maxillary sinus disease

Chart 2–14. **Head and Neck** (Figs. 2–30, 2–31)

Pathology	Ethmoid soft tissue lesion
Description	Differential could be papilloma involving nasal cavity, septum, and sinuses; benign lesion that infiltrates locally; biopsy needed
Symptoms	Asymptomatic until lesion is large enough to start obstructing nasal passages
Suggested protocols	Routine head, routine sinus
Appearance	Gray soft tissue component appears in area of sinuses, which should be black air filled; gray soft tissue invasion into white bone
Contrast	To enhance lesions

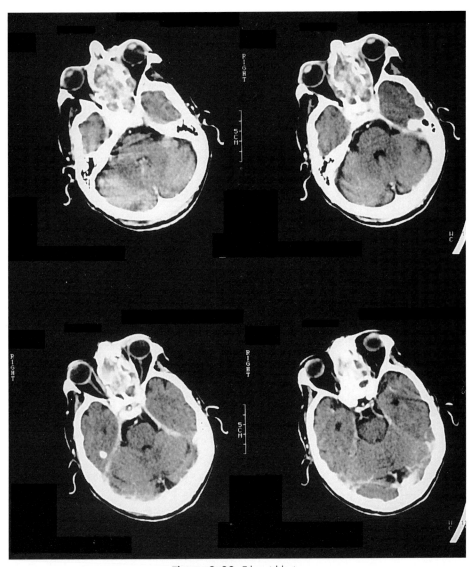

Figure 2–30. Ethmoid lesion

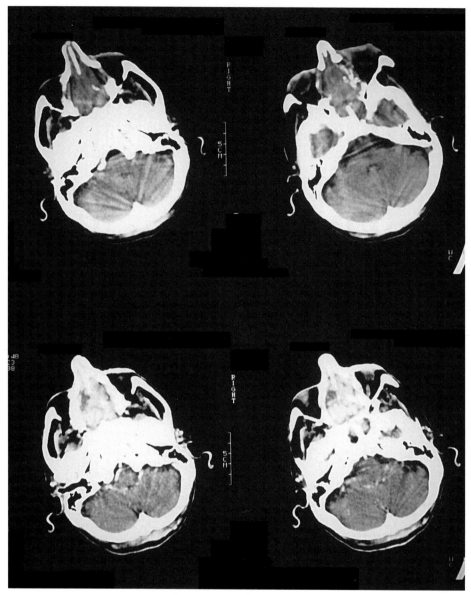

Figure 2-31. Ethmoid lesion

Chart 2–15. **Head and Neck** (Figs. 2–32, 2–33)

Pathology	Maxillary sinus lesion extending into ethmoid
Description	Differential could include a variety: papilloma (see ethmoid lesion), squamous cell carcinoma, which infiltrates extensively and metastasizes via lymph into cervical nodes; biopsy needed
Symptoms	Asymptomatic until large enough to cause congestion
Suggested protocols	Routine head, routine sinus
Appearance	Gray soft tissue appears as opposed to normal black air in maxillary sinus and ethmoid cells
Contrast	To enhance lesion

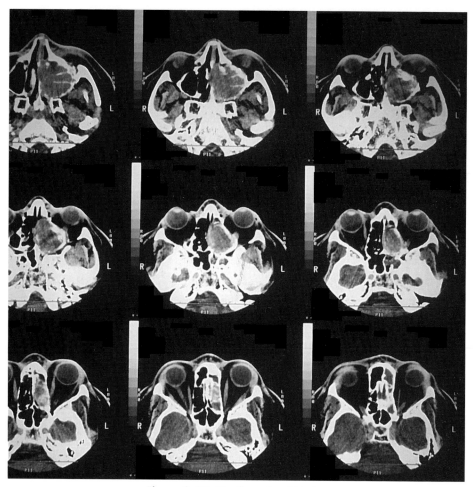

Figure 2–32. Maxillary-ethmoid lesion

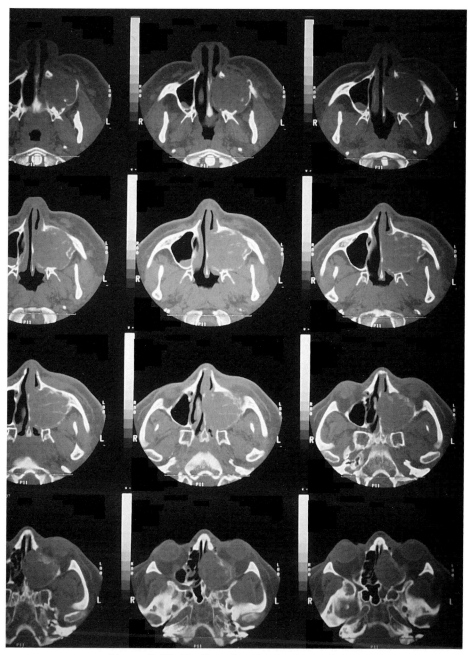

Figure 2–33. Maxillary-ethmoid lesion (bone window)

Chart 2–16. **Head and Neck** (Figs. 2–34 to 2–36)

Pathology	Tripod fracture of orbit Blow-out fracture of orbit
Description	Facial fracture with three components: zygomaticofrontal suture, zygomatic arch, and maxilla (anterior rim of orbit, lateral maxillary sinus) Blow-out fracture involves anterior portion of maxilla, creating "trap door" into maxillary sinus
Symptoms	Comes from a "punch" in the eye area Pain, swelling
Suggested protocols	Routine facial bones
Appearance	Soft tissue swelling, discontinuity of bone, dark irregular lines representing fracture
Contrast	Not necessary

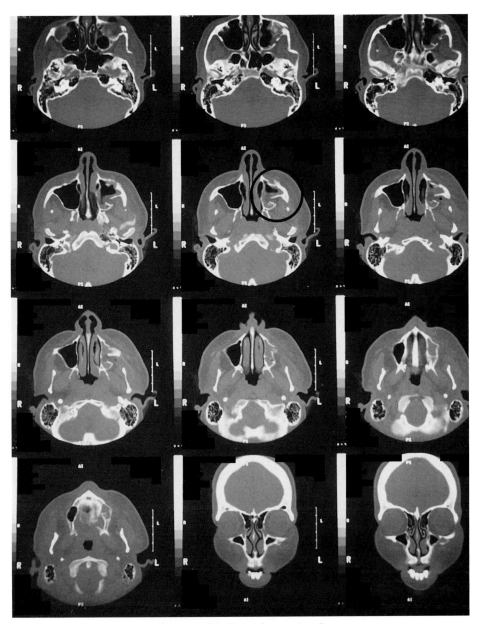

Figure 2–34. Tripod fracture (axial)

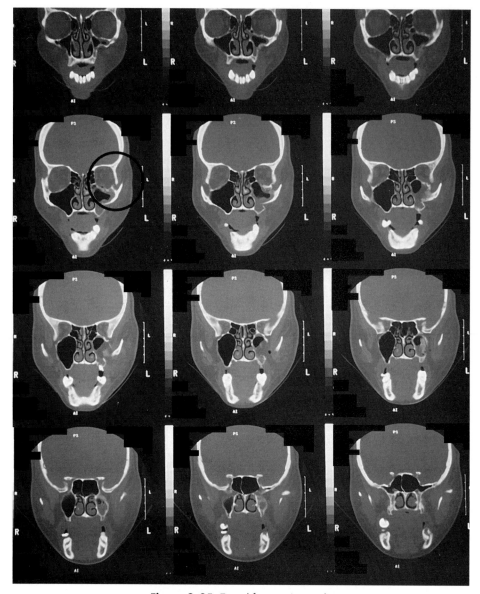

Figure 2–35. Tripod fracture (coronal)

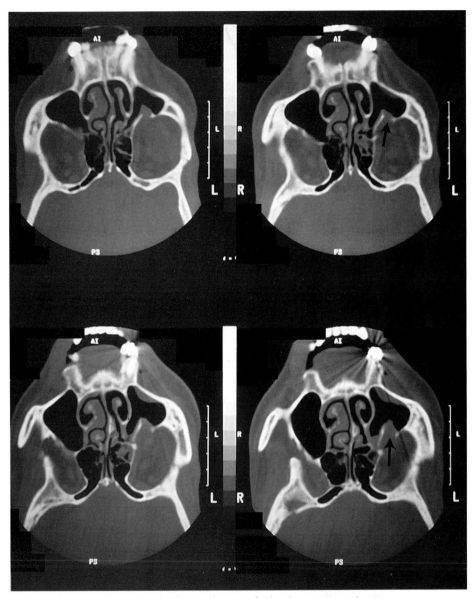

Figure 2–36. Blow-out fracture of orbit showing "trap door"

Chart 2–17. **Head and Neck** (Figs. 2–37, 2–38)

Pathology	Facial fractures from bullet penetration Invasion into neck with trauma
Description	Fractures of bone resulting from trauma to face and neck
Symptoms	Trauma
Suggested protocols	Routine facial bones using bone algorithm and bone window filming, with first scan starting inferior to check for cervical trauma
Appearance	Interruption of white facial bones: chips of white bone appear in the gray soft tissue area White streaks across cervical area from bullet on cervical slices
Contrast	Dependent on radiologist

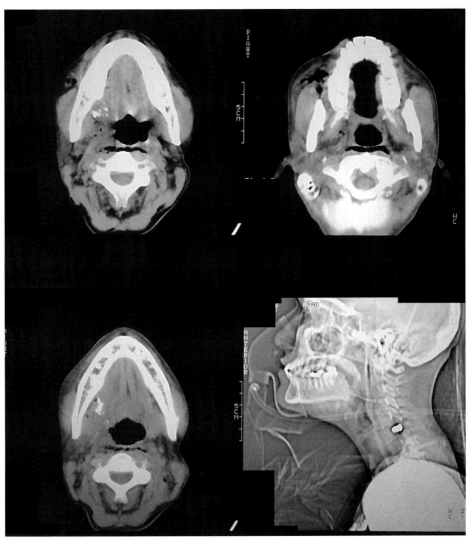

Figure 2–37. Facial fractures from bullet

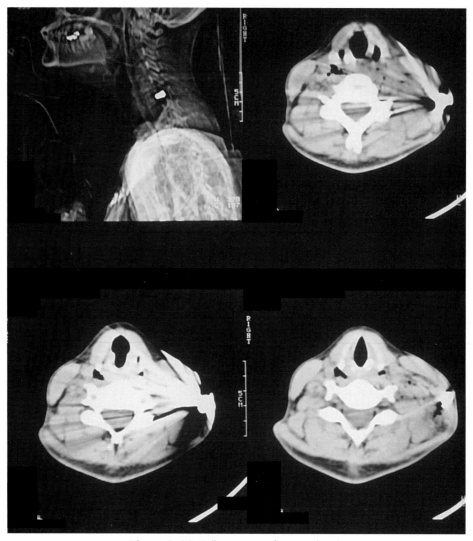

Figure 2–38. Bullet seen in soft tissue of neck

Chart 2–18. **Head and Neck** (Figs. 2–39 to 2–41)

Pathology	Parotid cyst, lesion
Description	Fluid-filled cysts in the parotid gland could be components of a more serious lesion
Symptoms	Fullness in area Pain around ear, problems with saliva production
Suggested protocols	Routine neck
Appearance	Fluid appears dark on CT
Contrast	To differentiate from other lesions

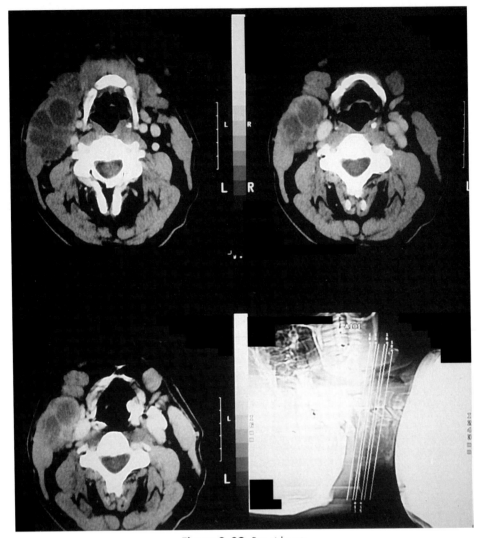

Figure 2-39. Parotid cysts

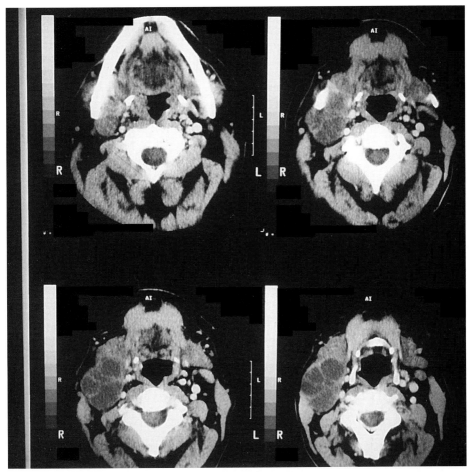

Figure 2–40. Parotid cysts

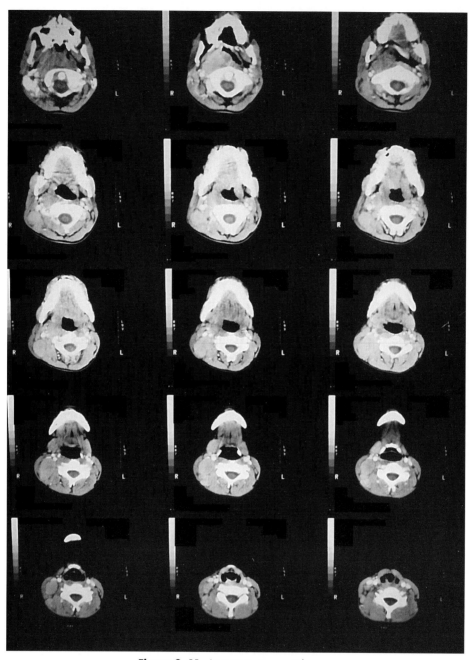

Figure 2–41. Asymmetry in parotid areas

Chart 2–19. **Head and Neck** (Figs. 2–42 to 2–44)

Pathology	Neck cancer
Description	Differential could be lymphoma, which is nodular or ulcerative in nature, resembling a carcinoma, or squamous cell carcinoma in which squamous cells grow abnormally and progress to cancer with ulcerations
Symptoms	Hoarseness, persistent sore throat, difficulty speaking
Suggested protocols	Routine neck
Appearance	Lesion appears gray with some necrotic (black) components pushing aside normal structures such as the trachea
Contrast	To enhance lesion

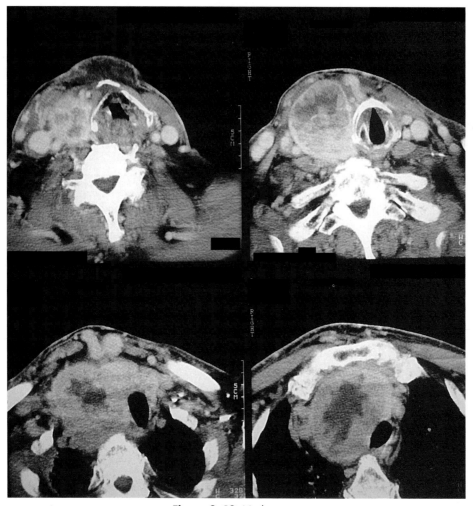

Figure 2–42. Neck cancer

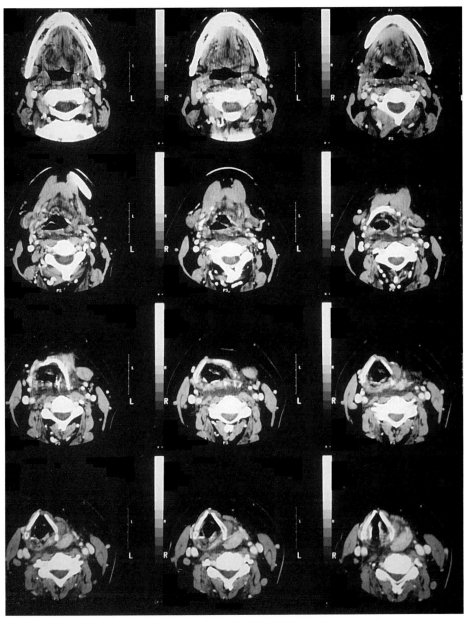

Figure 2–43. Lesion in neck

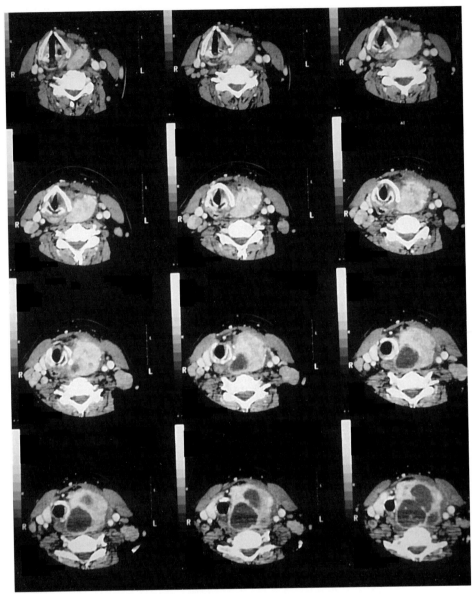

Figure 2–44. Lesion in neck

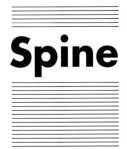

CHAPTER THREE

Spine

Chart 3–1. **Spine** (Fig. 3–1)

Pathology	Lumbar vertebral body fracture
Description	A break or disruption in the bone or cartilage as a result of trauma
Symptoms	Back pain
Suggested protocols	Routine lumbar
Appearance	Dark, irregular lines through white trabecular bone of vertebral body
Contrast	Dependent on radiologist

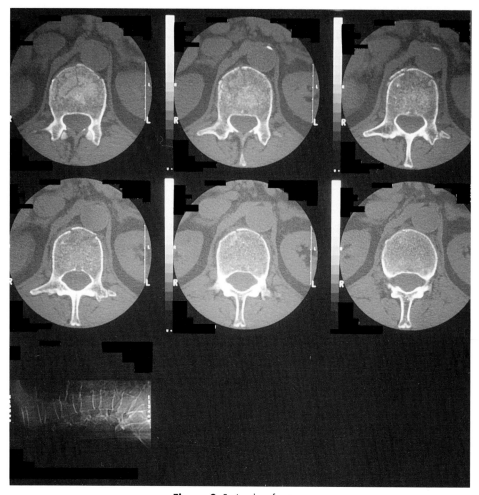

Figure 3–1. Lumbar fracture

Chart 3–2. **Spine** (Fig. 3–2)

Pathology	Cervical fracture
Description	A break or disruption in bone or cartilage as a result of trauma
Symptoms	Neck pain
Suggested protocols	Routine cervical
Appearance	Bone is pushed into spinal canal; appearance is asymmetric from other side
Contrast	Dependent on radiologist

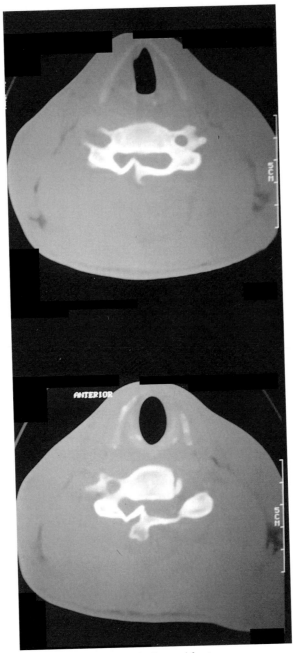

Figure 3–2. Cervical fracture

Chart 3–3. **Spine** (Figs. 3–3 to 3–5)

Pathology	Vacuum phenomenon
Description	Nitrogen (gas) forms in nucleus pulposus of disc as a result of degenerative changes in the tissue
Symptoms	Back pain
Suggested protocols	Routine lumbar
Appearance	Nucleus pulposus appears as a gray disc-shaped material with black air pockets interspersed in it
Contrast	Dependent on radiologist

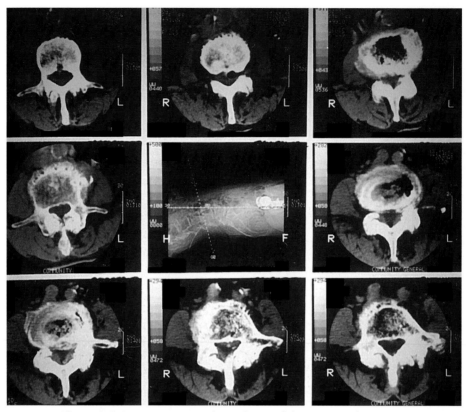

Figure 3-3. Nitrogen gas in nucleus pulposus of disc: vacuum phenomenon

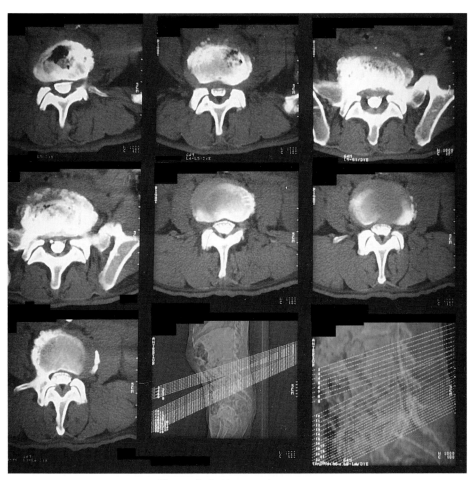

Figure 3–4. Vacuum phenomenon

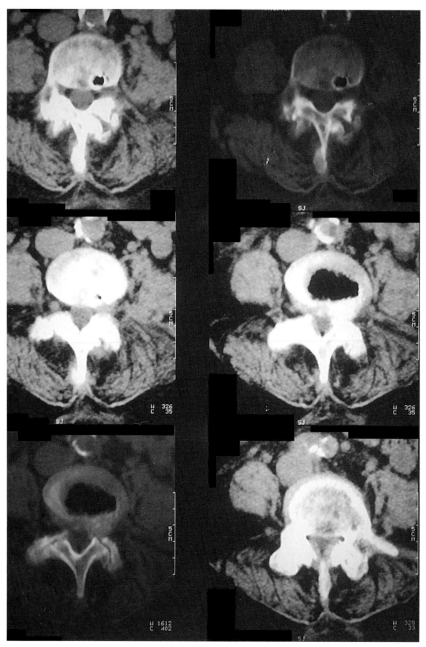

Figure 3–5. Vacuum phenomenon

Chart 3–4. **Spine** (Fig. 3–6)

Pathology	Lesion in sacrum
Description	Differential could include osteochondroma (a lesion that involves the spinous process; the margin of tumor is made of cortical bone with an inner, less dense component); giant cell tumor (usually benign but could progress into malignancy; usually involves the sacrum with cortical bone expansion with poorly defined margins), or chordoma (a common location is the sacrococcygeal region; appears as a lobulated mass arising in the bone and protruding into the spinal canal)
Symptoms	Back pain with radiation down legs
Suggested protocols	Routine lumbar
Appearance	On lumbar CTs, bone appears white, and lesion appears grayish in white bone; margins of bone are not visible, being hidden by lesion
Contrast	To enhance lesion in sacrum

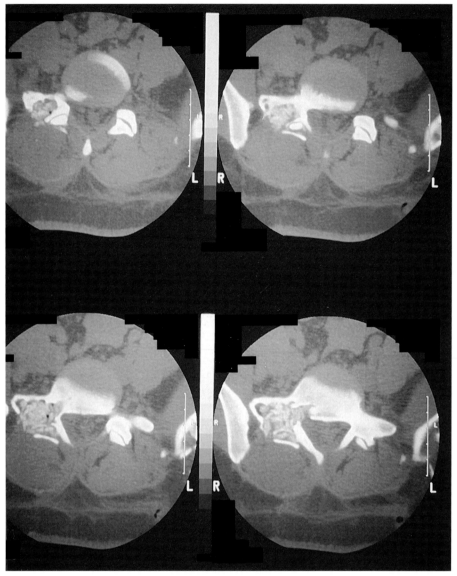

Figure 3–6. Sacral lesion

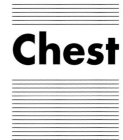

CHAPTER FOUR

Chest

Chart 4–1. **Chest** (Figs. 4–1 to 4–4)

Pathology	Lung lesion
Description	Lung cancers generally fall into two groups: central (bronchogenic) carcinoma (arises near the hilum of the lung) and peripheral carcinoma (arises in relation to the small bronchi, bronchioles, or alveoli; tends to be adenocarcinoma) The following fall under the two categories of lung cancer: large cell, small cell, squamous, adenocarcinomas, and alveolar cell; a biopsy is necessary to determine treatment regimen; common sites for metastases are adrenals, liver, brain, bone, and kidneys
Symptoms	Cough, hemoptysis, dyspnea, chest pain, weight loss
Suggested protocols	Routine chest
Appearance	Lesions appear gray in the black (air) lung field, thickening around vessels and hilum
Contrast	To differentiate vessels from adenopathy invasion

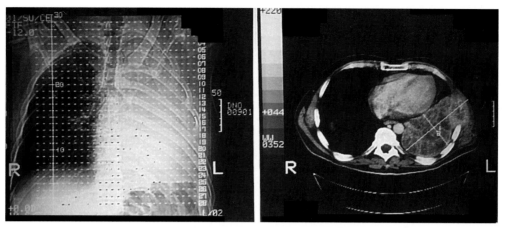

Figure 4–1. Left hemithorax lesion with invasion into ribs

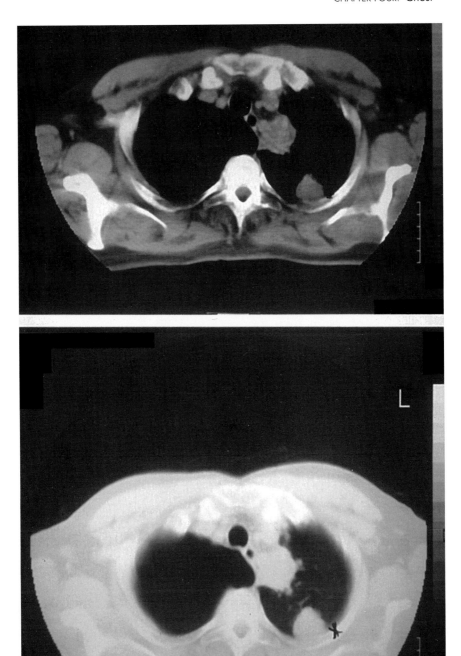

Figure 4–2. Left lung lesion

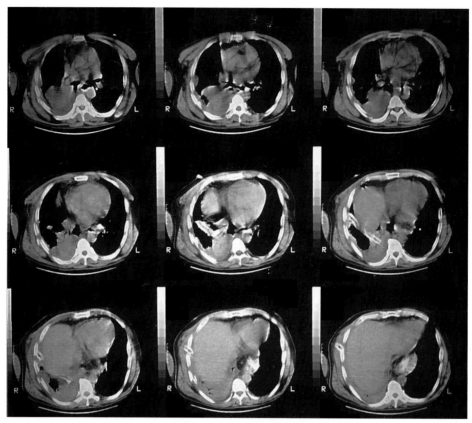

Figure 4–3. Right lung lesion

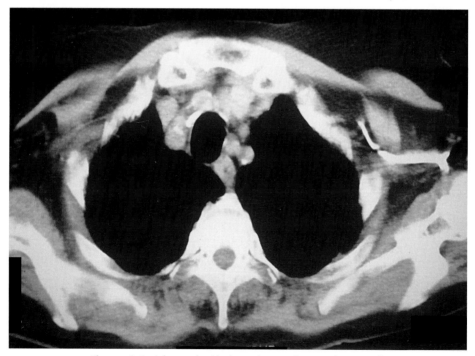

Figure 4–4. Adenopathy (thickening) around upper chest vessels

Chart 4–2. **Chest** (Fig. 4–5)

Pathology	Pneumothorax, rib fracture
Description	Presence of air in pleural cavity as a result of trauma; lung tissue collapses; air sucked into lung through chest wall defect
Symptoms	Acute onset of pain and dyspnea depending on size of pneumothorax
Suggested protocols	Routine chest
Appearance	No air in lung field; gray tissue of lung takes up space of black air in lung
Contrast	Dependent on radiologist

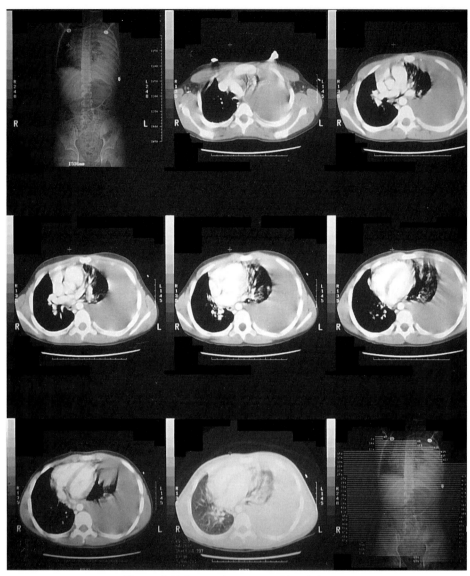

Figure 4–5. Pneumothorax caused by rib fracture

Chart 4–3. **Chest** (Fig. 4–6)

Pathology	Fibrous histiocytoma with fluid
Description	A granulomatous infiltration of interstitium by non-neoplastic histiocytes, common in young white males; disease regresses after a few months
Symptoms	Classically asymptomatic
Suggested protocols	Routine chest
Appearance	Cystic spaces with nodules occupying lung space as opposed to air
Contrast	To differentiate from cancerous lesions

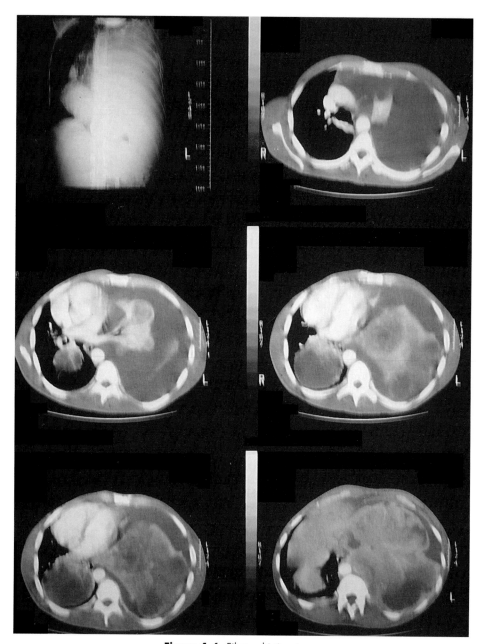

Figure 4–6. Fibrous histiocytoma

Chart 4–4. **Chest** (Figs. 4–7, 4–8)

Pathology	Lung abscess, empyema versus liver abscess
Description	Empyema of lung can occur as a result of acute or chronic bacterial pneumonia; area becomes walled off by fibrosis and filled with fluid
Symptoms	Low-grade fever, weight loss, productive cough
Suggested protocols	Routine chest
Appearance	Darker fluid-filled cavity in lung field
Contrast	To show active infectious process

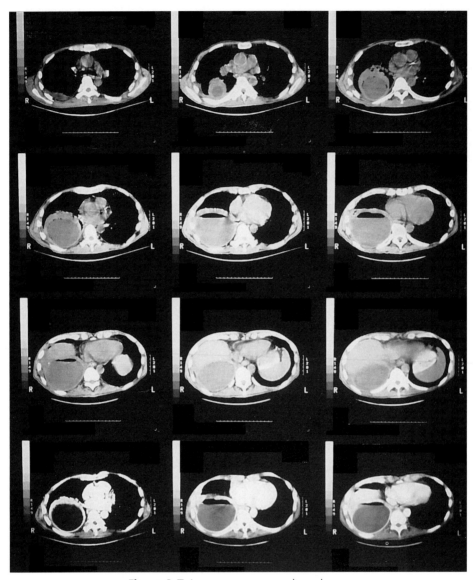

Figure 4–7. Lung empyema versus liver abscess

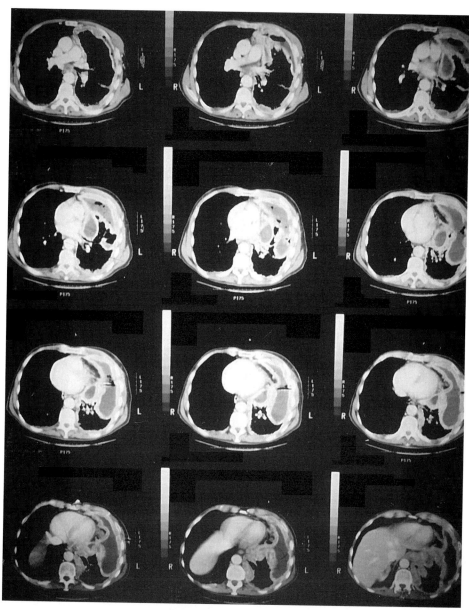

Figure 4–8. Lung abscess

Chart 4–5. **Chest** (Fig. 4–9)

Pathology	Stomach herniates to right side of chest cavity
Description	Stomach usually appears more inferiorly on left side of body; could be caused by surgical intervention
Symptoms	Reevaluation of surgical intervention
Suggested protocols	Routine chest and abdomen
Appearance	White (oral contrast) and gas (black) appear in base of right lung field
Contrast	Oral contrast for visualization of stomach Intravenous contrast dependent on radiologist

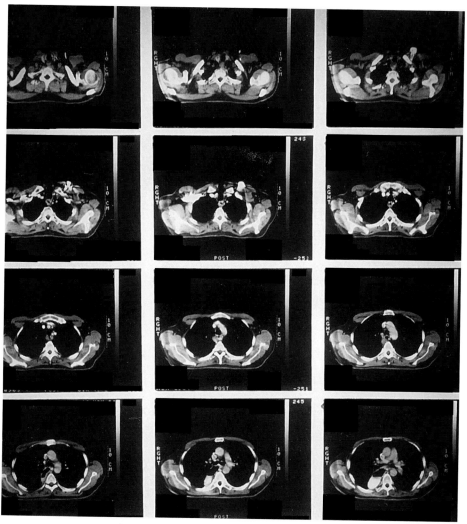

Figure 4–9. Stomach herniates to right chest cavity

Chart 4–6. Chest (Figs. 4–10, 4–11)

Pathology	Left brachiocephalic vein thrombus
Description	Formed from different components of blood (platelets, red blood cells, white blood cells); can be attached to vessel wall without causing complete obstruction of vessel flow; can be due to sluggish blood flow from diseases such as atherosclerosis or inflammation
Symptoms	Poor circulation, edema in upper extremities
Suggested protocols	Routine chest
Appearance	Left shoulder area appears to be full of "buckshot" but actually bright intravenous contrast in collateral circulation formed because of thrombus
Contrast	To help visualize vessels and thrombus

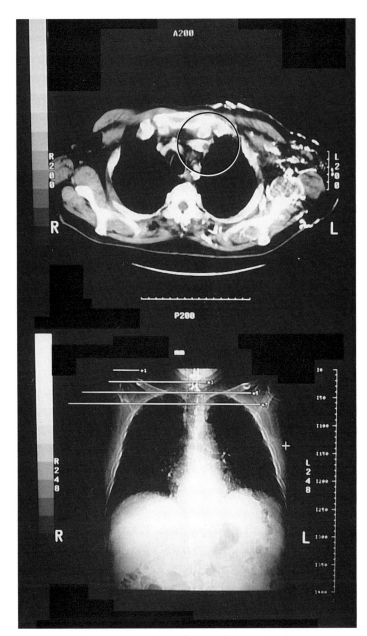

Figure 4–10. Left brachiocephalic vein thrombus

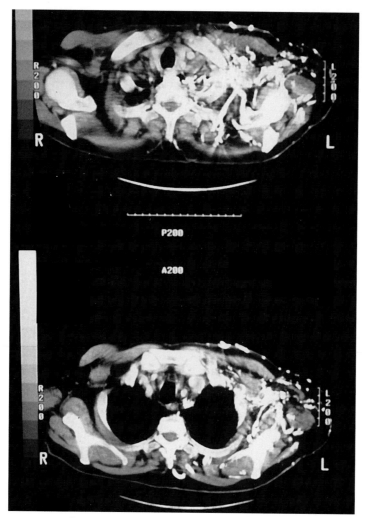

Figure 4–11. Buckshot appearance from thrombus

Chart 4–7. **Chest** (Figs. 4–12 to 4–14)

Pathology	Aortic dissection
Description	Disruption of media of aorta by entry of blood under high pressure through intimal tear usually caused by hypertension; occurs just above aortic valve or just distal to ligamentum arteriosum; blood dissects between layers of smooth muscles
Symptoms	Sudden onset of severe pain in chest; mimics heart attack; if ruptures, causes massive hemorrhage
Suggested protocols	Routine chest
Appearance	Dark irregular line in lumen of aorta representing split or dissection
Contrast	To visualize specific area of dissection

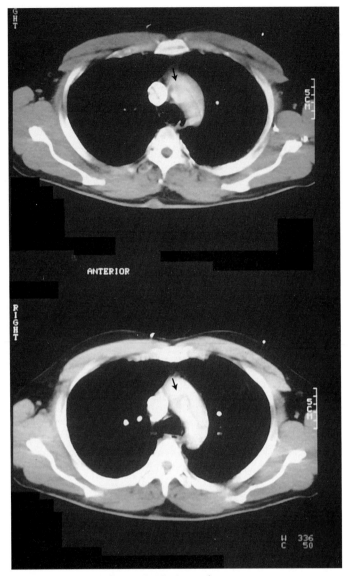

Figure 4–12. Aortic dissection

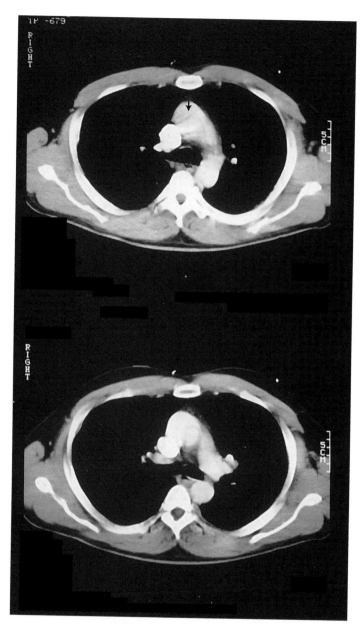

Figure 4–13. Aortic dissection

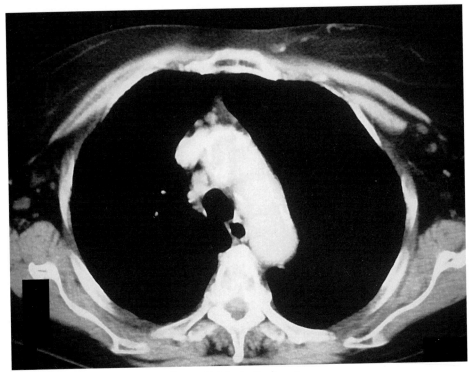

Figure 4-14. Aortic dissection

Chart 4–8. **Chest** (Figs. 4–15 to 4–17)

Pathology	Aortic aneurysm
Description	With severe atherosclerotic disease in aorta, a weakened wall will dilate and appear as the whole vessel enlarged or a saccular bulge on one side
Symptoms	Chest pain, increased blood pressure
Suggested protocols	Routine chest and abdomen
Appearance	Vessel appears larger than normal diameter or bulging on one side
Contrast	To better visualize vessels

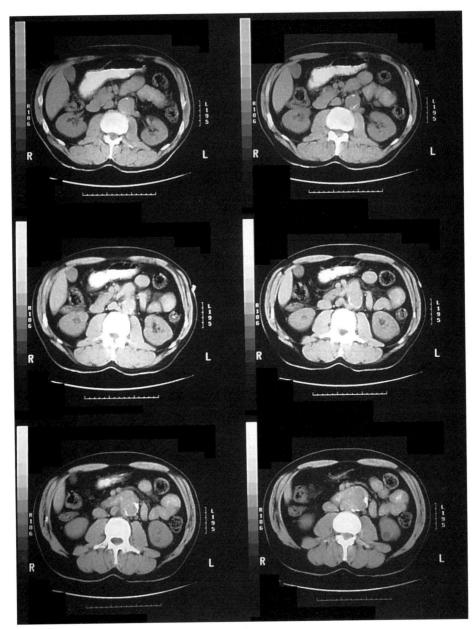

Figure 4–15. Aortic aneurysm

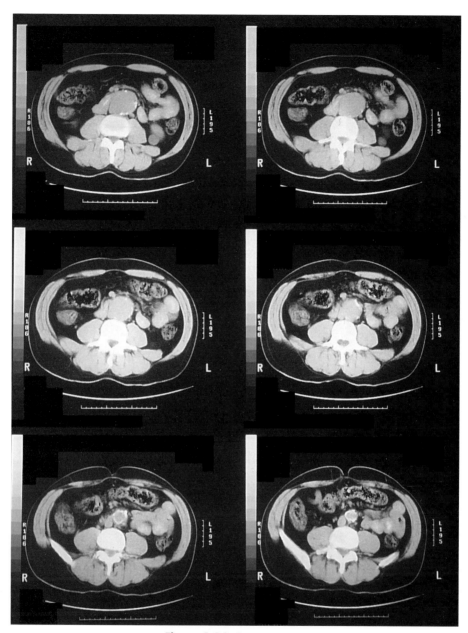

Figure 4-16. Aortic aneurysm

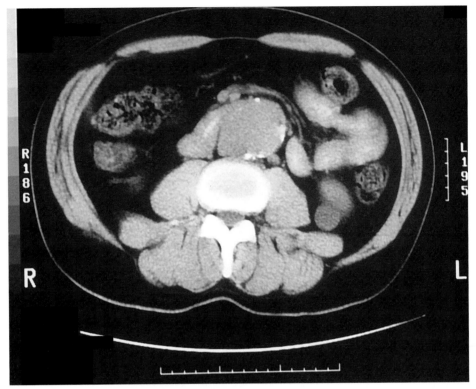

Figure 4–17. Aortic aneurysm

CHAPTER FIVE

Abdomen and Pelvis

Chart 5–1. **Abdomen and Pelvis** (Fig. 5–1)	
Pathology	Stomach lesion
Description	Metastatic lesion from melanoma involving the gastric mucosa
Symptoms	History of melanoma Stomach pain with digestive problems
Suggested protocols	Routine chest and abdomen
Appearance	Lesion appears as an irregularity of stomach wall
Contrast	Oral contrast to highlight stomach and bowel Intravenous contrast dependent on radiologist

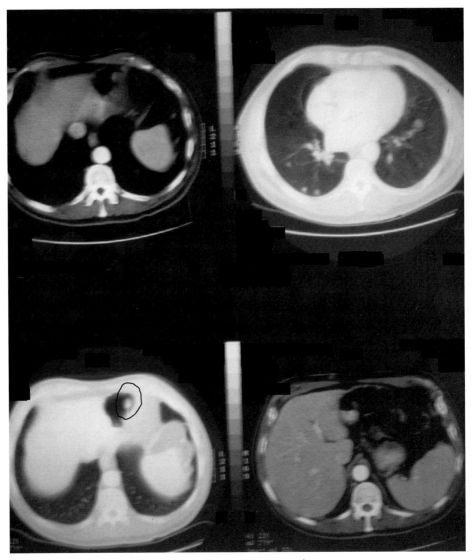

Figure 5-1. Lesion in stomach

Chart 5–2. **Abdomen and Pelvis** (Figs. 5–2, 5–3)

Pathology	Pancreatic head lesion, retroperitoneal sarcoma
Description	Lesion in the pancreas of connective tissue, highly malignant, proliferation of mesodermal cells
Symptoms	Could have common bile duct obstruction, anemia, weight loss
Suggested protocols	Routine abdomen
Appearance	Gray pancreas has mixed attenuations (darker-lighter) with irregular borders
Contrast	Oral contrast to highlight gastrointestinal tract Intravenous contrast to enhance lesions

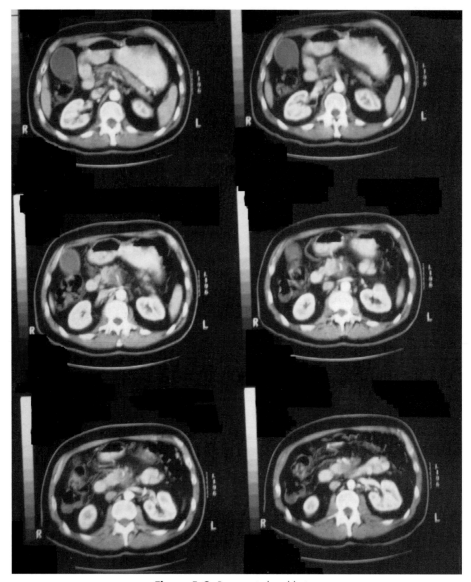

Figure 5–2. Pancreatic head lesion

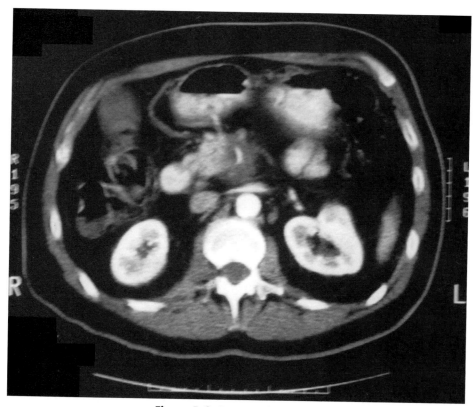

Figure 5-3. Pancreatic head lesion

Chart 5–3. **Abdomen and Pelvis** (Fig. 5–4)

Pathology	Retroperitoneal lymphoma
Description	Could be primary malignant lymphoma occurring as solid lesion; differential includes metastases; determination difficult unless patient has a history of cancer
Symptoms	Fatigue, flank pain, fullness in abdomen
Suggested protocols	Routine abdomen
Appearance	Small, gray lymph nodes around spine are large; lesions displace other structures
Contrast	Oral contrast to highlight gastrointestinal tract Intravenous contrast to differentiate structures and vasculature

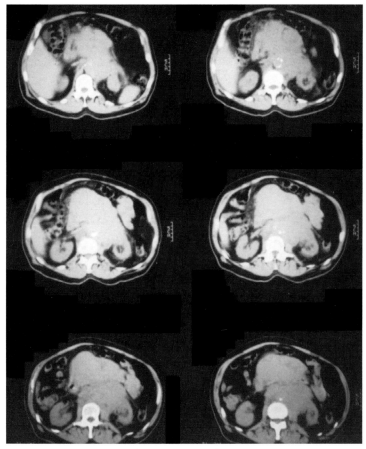

Figure 5–4. Lymphoma

Chart 5–4. **Abdomen and Pelvis** (Figs. 5–5, 5–6)

Pathology	Adrenal cyst, lesion Spine metastasis
Description	Lesion to adrenal is common for metastases from lung, breast, colon, and melanoma Cyst is fluid filled; adrenal cyst is less common than a renal cyst Spine metastasis was found by chance; cancer cells have invaded bone and changed attenuation of tissue
Symptoms	Known primary cancer, hormone imbalance, back pain
Suggested protocols	Routine abdomen
Appearance	Adrenal gland should appear as a small, y-shaped gray area superior to kidney; lesion enlarges gland as does the dark fluid-filled cyst; metastasis to the spine is dark appearing next to whiter bone
Contrast	To enhance lesions

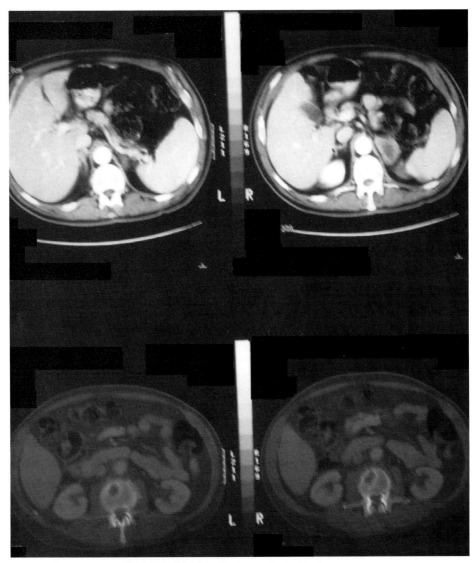

Figure 5–5. Adrenal metastases, spinal metastases

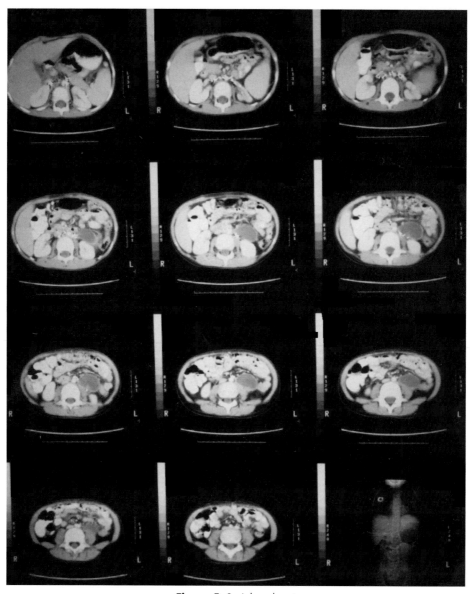

Figure 5–6. Adrenal cyst

Chart 5–5. **Abdomen and Pelvis** (Figs. 5–7 to 5–11)

Pathology	Ascites: abdominal and pelvic
Description	Serous fluid, which accumulates in peritoneal cavity as a result of imbalance of osmotic-pressure forces
Symptoms	Portal hypertension, fullness in abdomen, decrease in serum albumin levels
Suggested protocols	Routine abdomen
Appearance	Fluid appears darker around lighter gray liver
Contrast	Oral to highlight gastrointestinal tract Intravenous contrast to see vessels and lesions

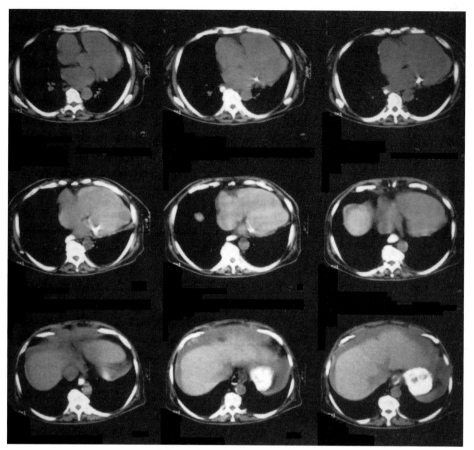

Figure 5–7. Ascites around liver

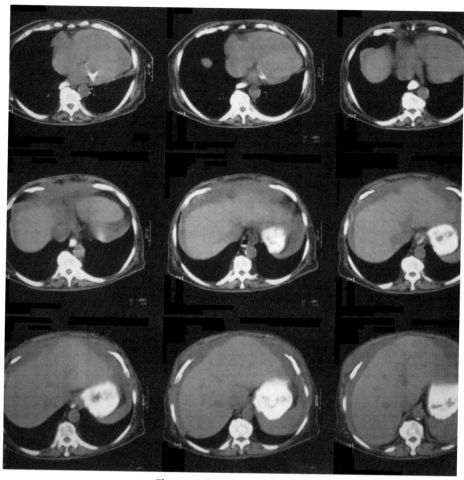

Figure 5–8. Ascites around liver

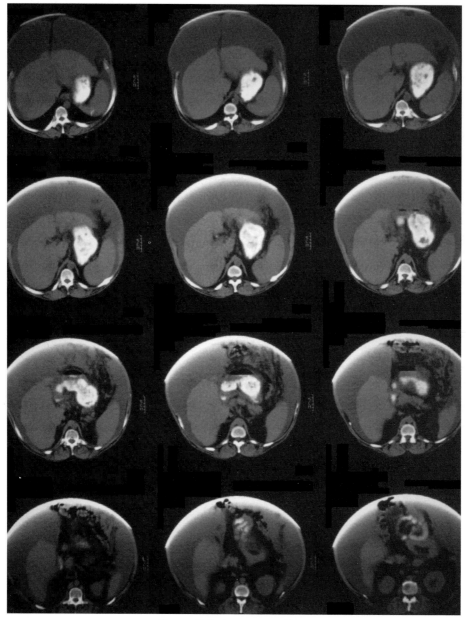

Figure 5–9. Ascites around liver

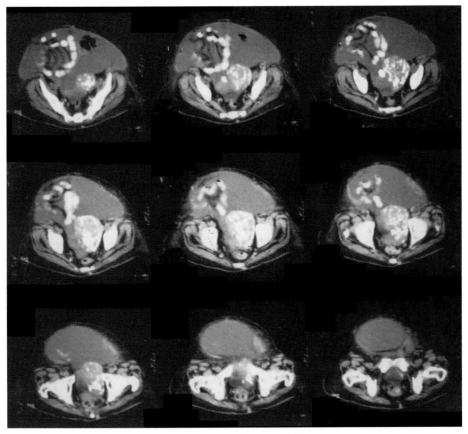

Figure 5–10. Ascites in pelvis

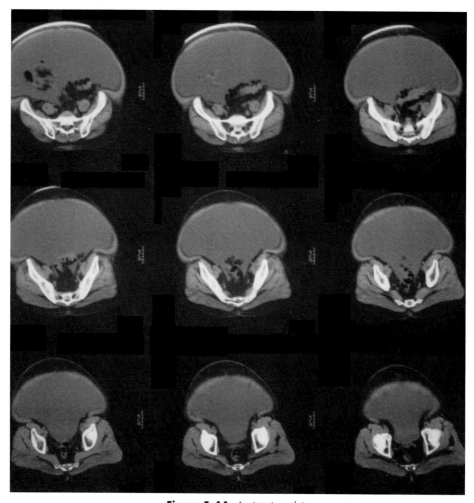

Figure 5-11. Ascites in pelvis

Chart 5–6. **Abdomen and Pelvis** (Figs. 5–12 to 5–14)

Pathology	Liver metastasis
Description	Most cancers from gastrointestinal tract, lung, breast, and melanomas travel to the liver; lesions often contain necrotic (dark) components
Symptoms	History of primary cancer Liver enlargement
Suggested protocols	Routine abdomen
Appearance	Lesions show up dark against the bright liver immediately after contrast injection; lesions become isodense with liver and cannot be visualized if scanning process is delayed
Contrast	Oral contrast to highlight gastrointestinal tract Intravenous contrast to detect liver lesions

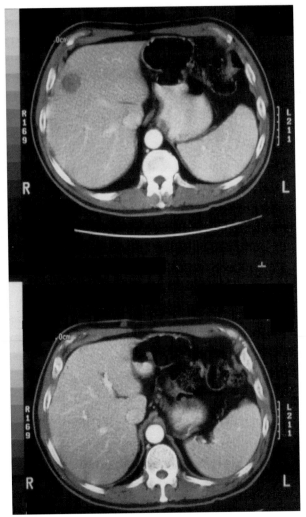

Figure 5–12. Liver metastases in right lobe

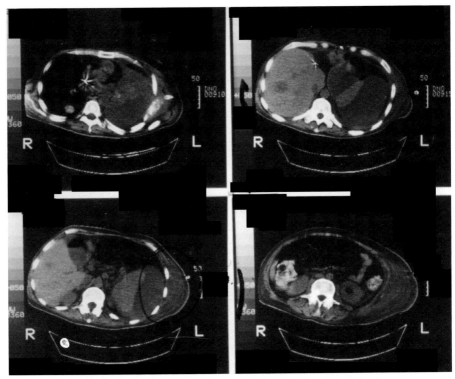

Figure 5-13. Liver metastases with chest tube infection on left side

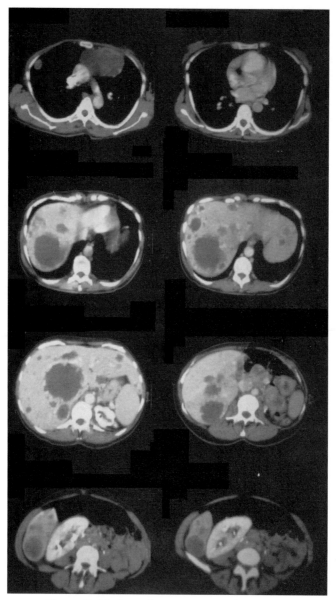

Figure 5-14. Severe liver metastases or liver cancer

Chart 5–7. **Abdomen and Pelvis** (Figs. 5–15, 5–16)

Pathology	Liver laceration
Description	Tearing of liver tissue as a result of trauma; bleeding from disruption of small or large blood vessels
Symptoms	Right-sided pain; trauma to liver area, lowering blood count
Suggested protocols	Routine abdomen
Appearance	Discontinuity of gray liver, almost like a fracture in a bone; dark fluid around tear
Contrast	Dependent on radiologist

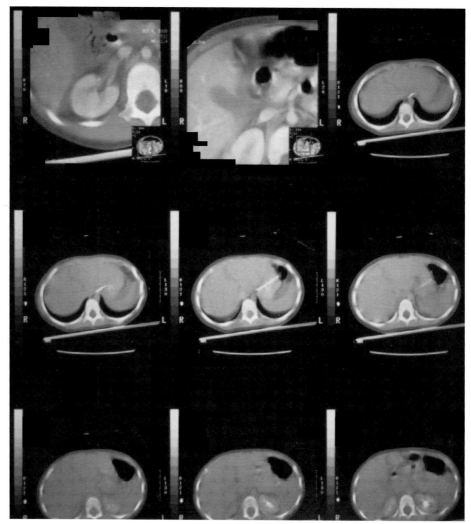

Figure 5-15. Liver laceration

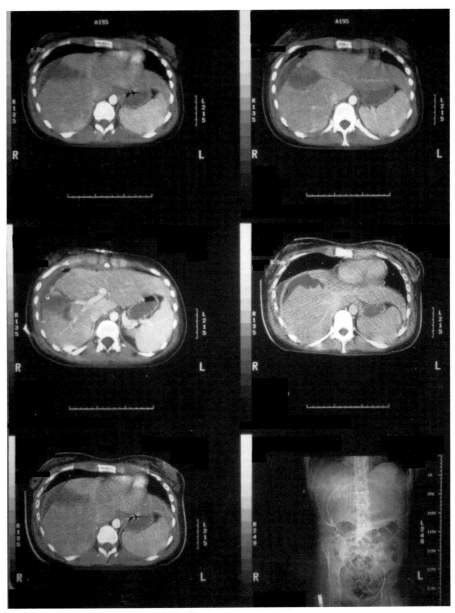

Figure 5-16. Liver laceration

Chart 5–8. **Abdomen and Pelvis** (Fig. 5–17)

Pathology	Spleen laceration
Description	Tearing of splenic tissue as a result of trauma; bleeding in area from disruption of small or large blood vessels
Symptoms	Left-sided pain
Suggested protocols	Routine abdomen
Appearance	Discontinuity of gray spleen, almost like a bone fracture; dark fluid around tear
Contrast	Dependent on radiologist

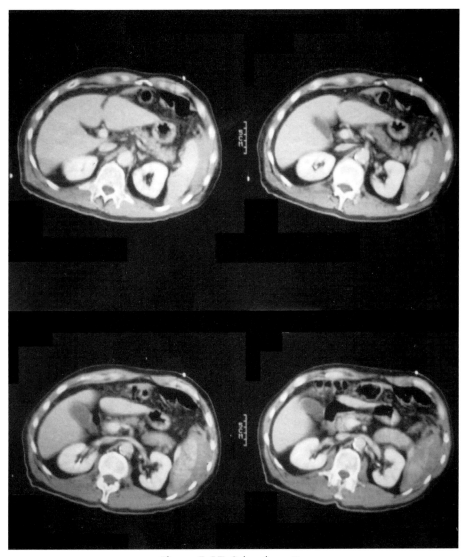

Figure 5-17. Spleen laceration

Chart 5-9. **Abdomen and Pelvis** (Fig. 5-18)

Pathology	Infarcted spleen
Description	Ischemic because of insufficient arterial blood supply or venous outflow; results in necrosis of tissue
Symptoms	Pain
Suggested protocols	Routine abdomen
Appearance	Spleen appears dark because of infarction instead of normal gray
Contrast	Oral contrast to highlight gastrointestinal tract Intravenous contrast to enhance lesions

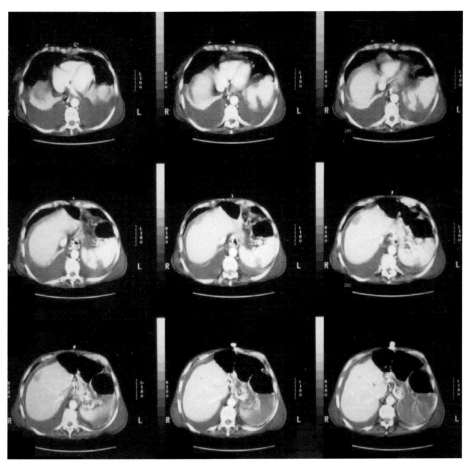

Figure 5-18. Infarcted spleen

Chart 5–10. **Abdomen and Pelvis** (Fig. 5–19)

Pathology	Renal cortex variant with "cauliflower" appearance
Description	Anomaly in which kidney cortex has flower petal appearance
Symptoms	Asymptomatic or kidney function problems
Suggested protocols	Routine abdomen
Appearance	Cortex of kidney has flower petal appearance
Contrast	To check for good kidney function

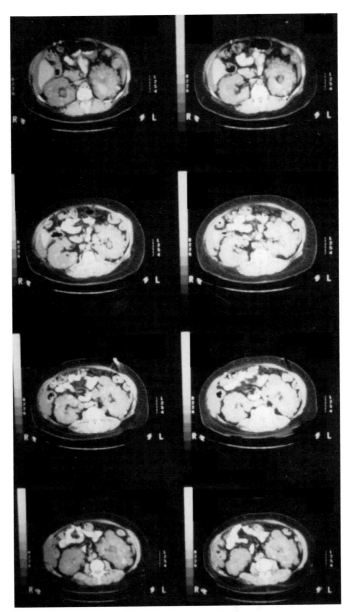

Figure 5–19. Kidneys with renal cortex variant

Chart 5–11. **Abdomen and Pelvis** (Fig. 5–20)

Pathology	Necrotic kidney with abscess
Description	Probable coagulative necrosis (cells retain cellular outline), usually as a result of deficient blood supply Abscess forms because of infection in the necrotic tissue; has extended through the renal capsule into the perirenal fat
Symptoms	Pain with urination, flank pain
Suggested protocols	Routine abdomen
Appearance	Necrotic cells appear dark
Contrast	Dependent on radiologist and laboratory work

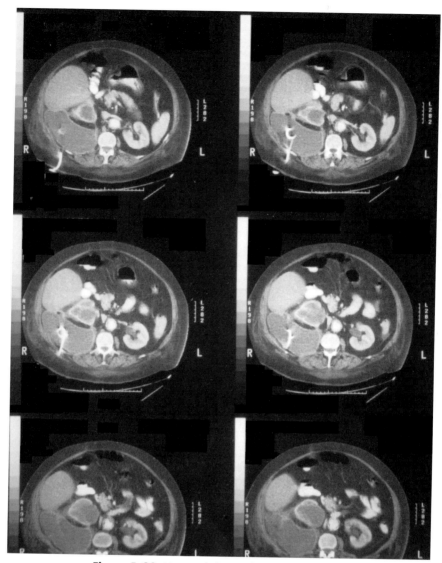

Figure 5-20. Necrotic kidney with subsequent abscess

Chart 5–12. **Abdomen and Pelvis** (Figs. 5–21, 5–22)

Pathology	Cyst in right kidney Left kidney infarcted because of thrombus in renal vein
Description	Cysts present in more than 50% of patients older than 50 years Infarcted kidney from ischemia caused by thrombus in renal vein
Symptoms	Onset of flank pain, hematuria
Suggested protocols	Routine abdomen
Appearance	Kidney is dark from infarction; thrombus in vein appears as a dark, filling defect
Contrast	Oral contrast to highlight gastrointestinal tract Intravenous contrast to visualize thrombus in vein

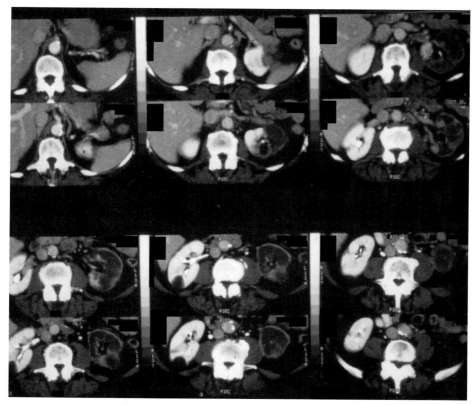

Figure 5–21. Right kidney cyst, infarcted left kidney

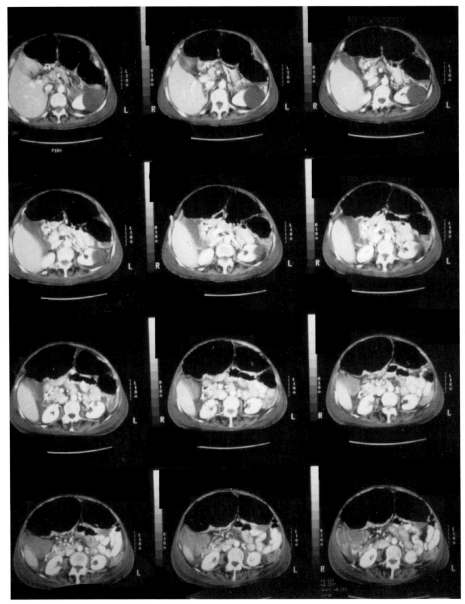

Figure 5–22. Left kidney cyst

Chart 5–13. **Abdomen and Pelvis** (Fig. 5–23)

Pathology	Cystic nephroma
Description	1- to 10-mm cystic lesion not projecting beyond cortical margin of kidney; arises from neural tissue; occurs in pediatric cases
Symptoms	Fullness in abdomen, kidney dysfunction
Suggested protocols	Routine abdomen
Appearance	Lesion appears as a large, dark, fluid-filled cavity
Contrast	Intravenous contrast to differentiate from solid lesion

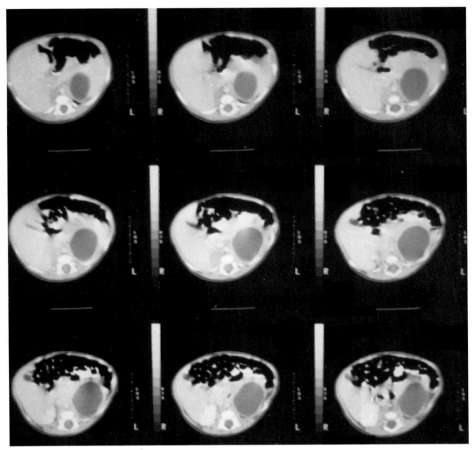

Figure 5–23. Cystic nephroma

Chart 5–14. **Abdomen and Pelvis** (Fig. 5–24)

Pathology	Atrophied kidneys
Description	Kidneys are not functional because of disease process or congenital abnormalities; kidney transplant needed
Symptoms	Kidney function poor or nonexistent; chronic renal failure
Suggested protocols	Routine abdomen
Appearance	Kidneys are extremely small gray structures
Contrast	Dependent on radiologist

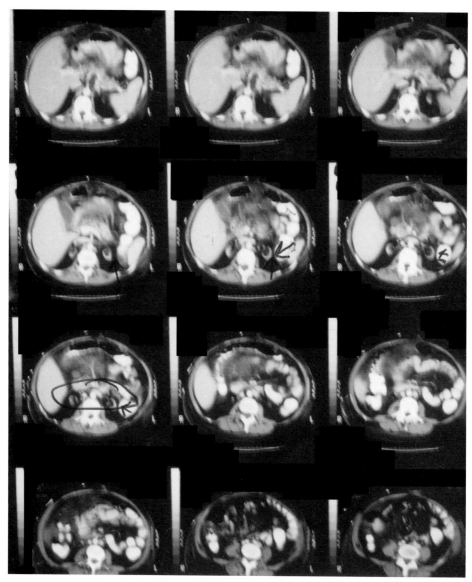

Figure 5–24. Atrophied kidneys

Chart 5–15. **Abdomen and Pelvis** (Fig. 5–25)

Pathology	Transplanted kidney
Description	Donor kidney is placed in the pelvic region to take over for the atrophied kidneys
Symptoms	Postsurgical recheck for function and appearance
Suggested protocols	Routine abdomen and pelvis
Appearance	Transplanted kidney is located in the pelvis
Contrast	Intravenous contrast to check for function

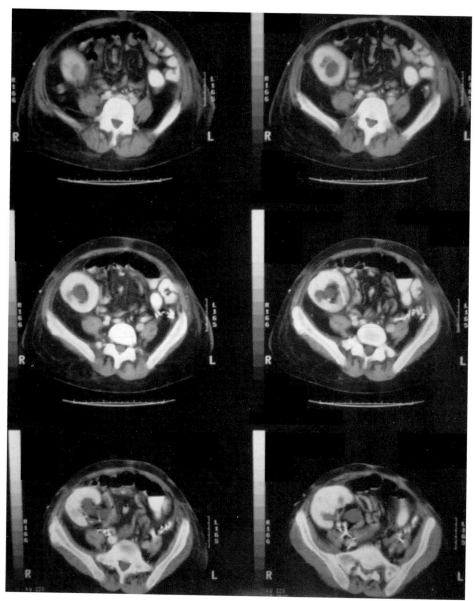

Figure 5–25. Transplanted kidney

Chart 5–16. **Abdomen and Pelvis** (Fig. 5–26)

Pathology	Renal cell carcinoma with invasion into inferior vena cava
Description	Solid, encapsulated, necrotic lesion from epithelial cells; most common malignant lesion of kidney; can be small to massive in size; rarely infiltrates into fascia, but can invade the renal vein and extend into the inferior vena cava; metastasizes to lung, bone, and brain
Symptoms	Flank pain, hematuria, fever, anemia
Suggested protocols	Routine abdomen and pelvis
Appearance	Lesion appears darker than normal kidney, large in size, as infiltrates into renal vein and then inferior vena cava; appears as a dark, filling defect in the vessel
Contrast	Oral contrast to highlight gastrointestinal tract Intravenous contrast to enhance metastasis and visualize invasion process into vessels

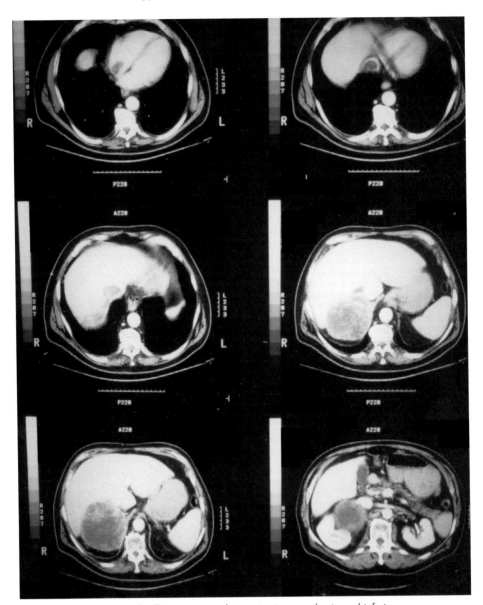

Figure 5–26. Renal cell carcinoma with invasion into renal vein and inferior vena cava

Chart 5–17. **Abdomen and Pelvis** (Fig. 5–27)

Pathology	Inferior vena cava thrombus
Description	Thrombus is a formation of blood components (platelets, fibrin, red blood cells, white blood cells) attaching to the vessel wall but not obstructing; caused by sluggish flow from atherosclerotic disease
Symptoms	Chest pain, cardiac problems, lower extremity edema
Suggested protocols	Routine chest and abdomen
Appearance	Thrombus appears as a dark, filling defect in the normal lighter inferior vena cava
Contrast	Intravenous contrast for visualization of inferior vena cava and other vessels

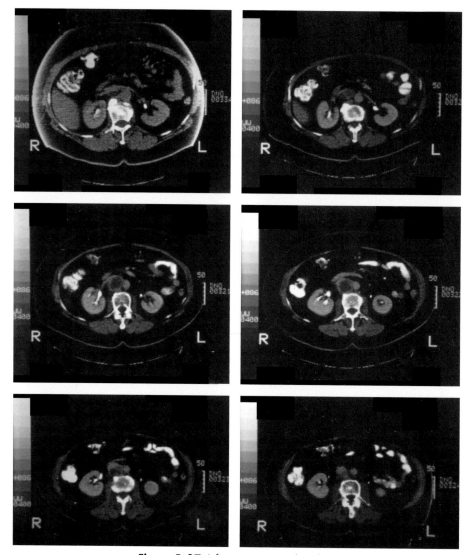

Figure 5–27. Inferior vena cava thrombus

Chart 5–18. **Abdomen and Pelvis** (Fig. 5–28)

Pathology	Ruptured mycotic aortic aneurysm
Description	Aneurysm (weakening and ballooning of wall of aorta) from infectious process, causing a slow hemorrhage into surrounding area
Symptoms	History of infection and other serious disease process, pain in abdomen
Suggested protocols	Routine chest, abdomen, and pelvis
Appearance	Increased size of aorta: fluid-filled cavity (darker) around vertebral body and aortic area
Contrast	Oral contrast to highlight gastrointestinal tract Intravenous contrast to show the asymmetries of aortic wall

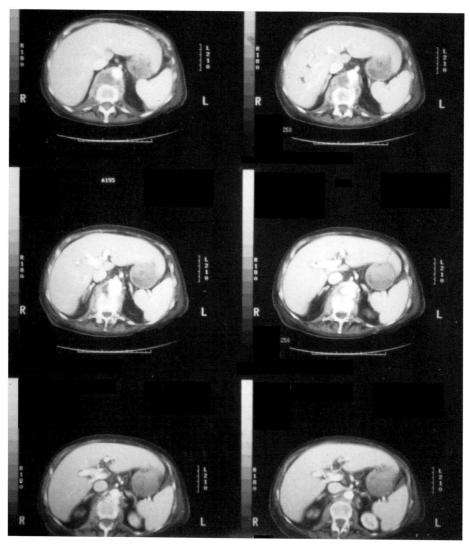

Figure 5-28. Ruptured mycotic aortic aneurysm

Chart 5–19. **Abdomen and Pelvis** (Fig. 5–29)

Pathology	Calcification of foreign body in subcutaneous tissue
Description	Foreign body lodged in subcutaneous tissue causes a reaction of the body of dystrophic calcification as a result of local abnormality in the tissue
Symptoms	Asymptomatic or pain in area
Suggested protocols	Routine abdomen
Appearance	Calcifications appear white in the gray subcutaneous tissue
Contrast	Oral contrast highlights gastrointestinal tract Intravenous contrast to differentiate from lesion

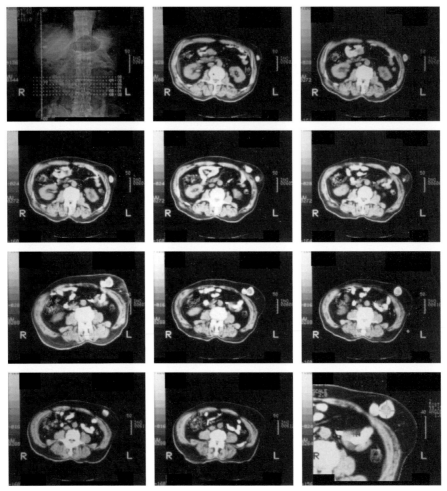

Figure 5–29. Calcification of foreign body in subcutaneous tissue

Chart 5–20. **Abdomen and Pelvis** (Fig. 5–30)

Pathology	Trauma pelvis with hematoma
Description	Localized extravasated blood occurring on right side, causing pressure or compression on ascending colon
Symptoms	Trauma, swelling in affected area, pain
Suggested protocols	Routine abdomen and pelvis
Appearance	Gray area asymmetric with other side of body; hematoma appears darker
Contrast	Dependent on radiologist

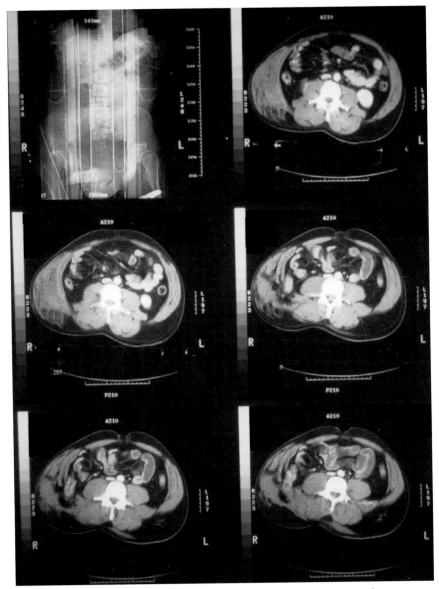

Figure 5–30. Hematoma affecting ascending colon in a trauma pelvis

Chart 5–21. **Abdomen and Pelvis** (Figs. 5–31, 5–32)

Pathology	Pelvic cyst
Description	Differentials could be ovarian cyst (darker fluid with lighter ring lining; smooth, regular borders), serous lesion of the ovary (filled with serous fluid; most benign, but some can be malignant or borderline), mesenteric cyst, seroma, and lymphocele
Symptoms	Heaviness in abdomen and pelvis
Suggested protocols	Routine abdomen and pelvis
Appearance	Dark fluid-filled cavity with lighter lining
Contrast	Oral contrast to highlight rectum and colon Intravenous contrast to highlight bladder

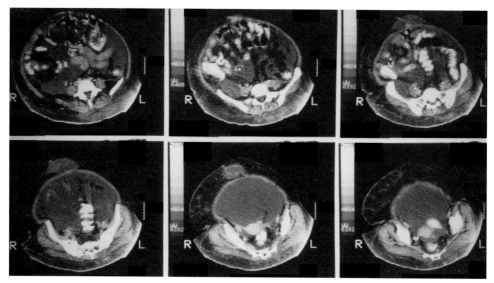

Figure 5–31. Pelvic cyst

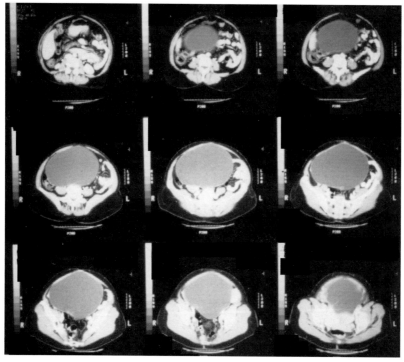

Figure 5–32. Pelvic cyst

Chart 5–22. **Abdomen and Pelvis** (Fig. 5–33)

Pathology	Pelvic lesion and cyst
Description	Differentials for pelvic lesion: retroperitoneal sarcoma (arises from connective tissue, highly malignant), adenopathy, and lymphoma
Symptoms	Heaviness in abdomen and pelvis; pain
Suggested protocols	Routine abdomen and pelvis
Appearance	Cysts appear dark with lighter and smooth borders Lesions have different attenuation, but not as dark as cysts; irregular margins
Contrast	Oral contrast to highlight rectum Intravenous contrast to highlight bladder

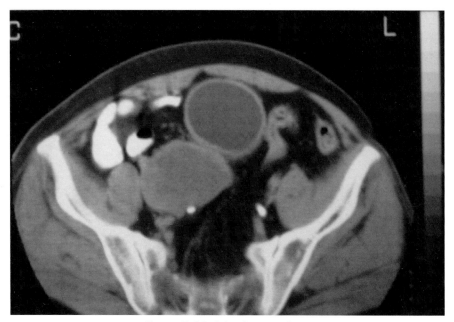

Figure 5–33. Pelvic lesion and cyst

Chart 5–23. **Abdomen and Pelvis** (Fig. 5–34)

Pathology	Hematoma from exploratory laparoscopic surgery
Description	Localized area of extravasated blood resulting from surgery; extends from surgical site inferiorly into the pelvis region
Symptoms	Temperature, pain, discomfort
Suggested protocols	Routine abdomen and pelvis
Appearance	Loculated area of blood (darker) displacing other structures in the abdominal and pelvic regions
Contrast	Oral contrast to highlight the gastrointestinal tract Intravenous contrast to differentiate from a lesion

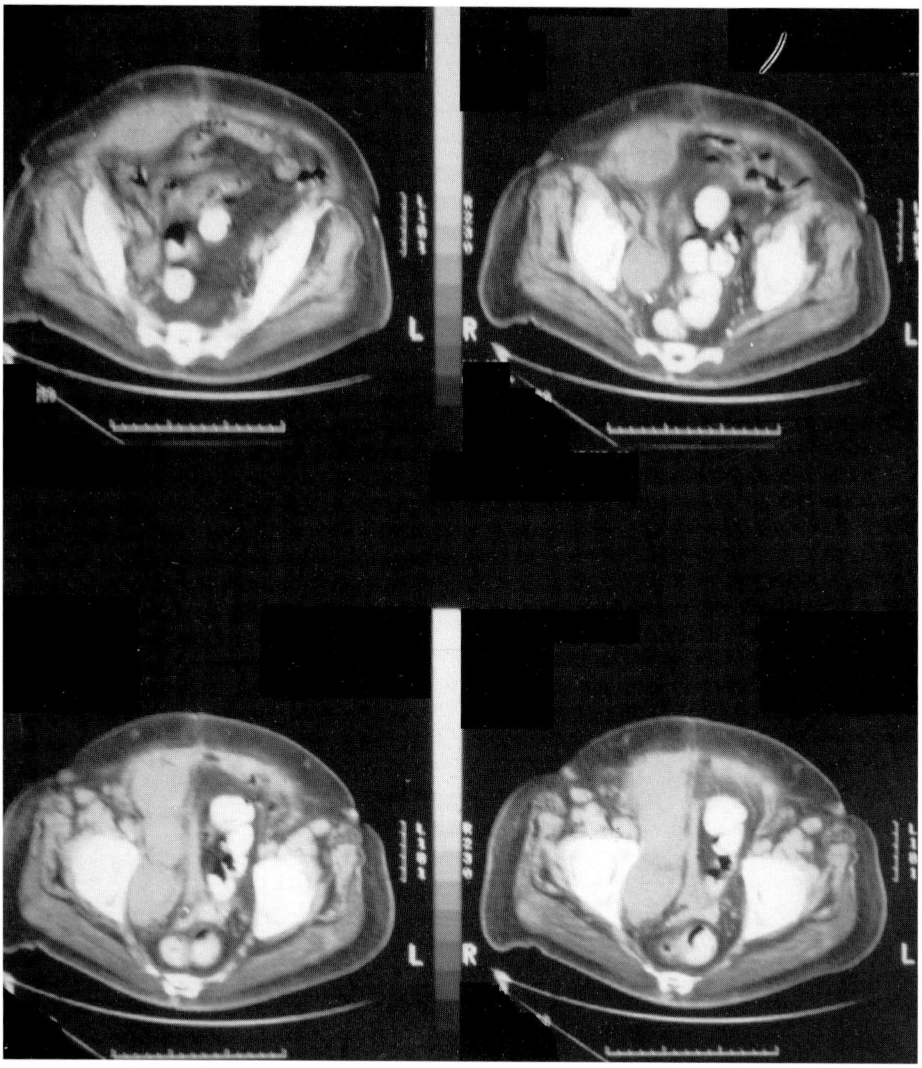

Figure 5–34. Hematoma from exploratory laparoscopic surgery

Chart 5–24. **Abdomen and Pelvis** (Fig. 5–35)

Pathology	Hernia
Description	Protrusion of a sac of peritoneum through a defect or weakness in the abdominal wall; sac may contain a variety of tissues such as omentum and bowel
Symptoms	Palpable through skin Weakened area; pain, pulling sensation
Suggested protocols	Routine abdomen and pelvis
Appearance	White oral contrast in bowel appears above the abdominal wall in the gray subcutaneous tissue
Contrast	Oral contrast to highlight gastrointestinal tract Intravenous contrast dependent on radiologist

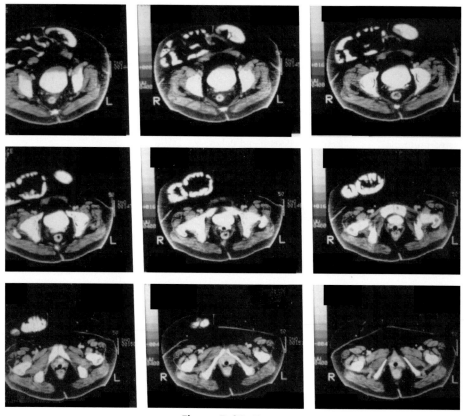

Figure 5–35. Hernia

Chart 5–25. **Abdomen and Pelvis** (Figs. 5–36, 5–37)

Pathology	Fistula between bladder–sigmoid colon area and vagina
Description	Abnormal pathway has formed connecting the bladder, vagina, and sigmoid colon; could be due to inflammatory process or cancer of cervix, colon, or bladder; can be associated with major infection
Symptoms	Dribbling of urine through vagina; passage of feces, gas, and urine through colon; air and fecal material through bladder
Suggested protocols	Routine abdomen and pelvis
Appearance	Abnormal gas in bladder; blending of feces, gas, and fluid in organs involved
Contrast	Oral contrast to highlight rectum and sigmoid Intravenous contrast to highlight bladder

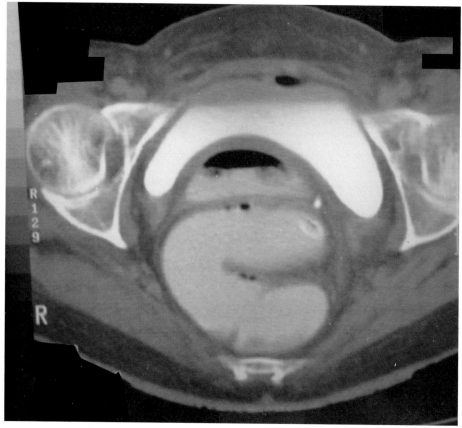

Figure 5–36. Fistula among bladder, sigmoid colon, and vagina

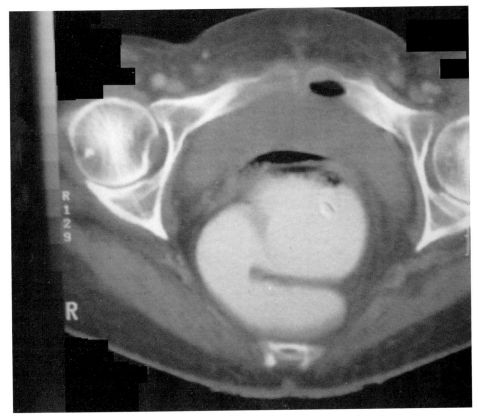

Figure 5–37. Fistula among bladder, sigmoid colon, and vagina

Chart 5–26. **Abdomen and Pelvis** (Figs. 5–38, 5–39)

Pathology	Rectal lesion
Description	Probable cancer of rectum; lesions are malignant ulcers with raised, everted edges
Symptoms	Asymptomatic in early stages Blood in stool with change in bowel habits
Suggested protocols	Routine abdomen and pelvis
Appearance	Rectum may appear larger, displacing bladder, uterus, or prostate
Contrast	Oral contrast to highlight rectum Intravenous contrast to highlight bladder Check for displacement

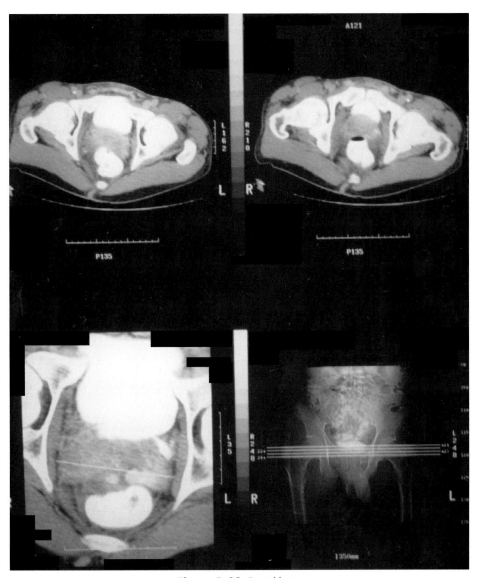

Figure 5–38. Rectal lesion

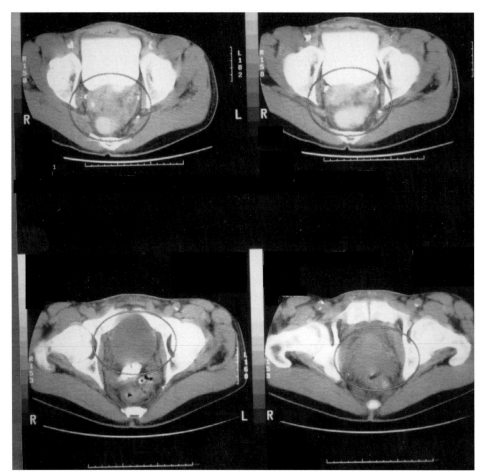

Figure 5–39. Rectal lesion

CHAPTER SIX

Musculoskeletal

Chart 6–1. **Musculoskeletal** (Fig. 6–1)

Pathology	Right iliac wing nonaggressive lesion
Description	Lesion could represent an osteochondroma, which is a benign lesion varying in size; usually occurs in the femur, tibia, and pelvis
Symptoms	Right hip pain, lower back pain
Suggested protocols	Routine pelvis using bone algorithm and 5-mm slice thickness
Appearance	With bone window filming, bone appears grayish with lesion appearing white
Contrast	To check for enhancement

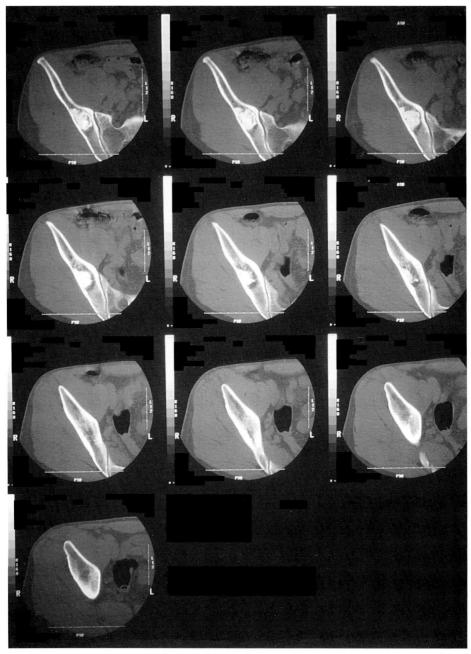

Figure 6–1. Right iliac wing lesion

Chart 6–2. **Musculoskeletal** (Fig. 6–2)

Pathology	Trauma pelvis with fractures
Description	Discontinuity of bones of pelvis with separation of iliac wing from sacral body
Symptoms	Trauma
Suggested protocols	Routine pelvis to check for organ damage Reconstructions with bone algorithm for fractures
Appearance	Fractures appear as dark irregularities in bone
Contrast	Dependent on radiologist

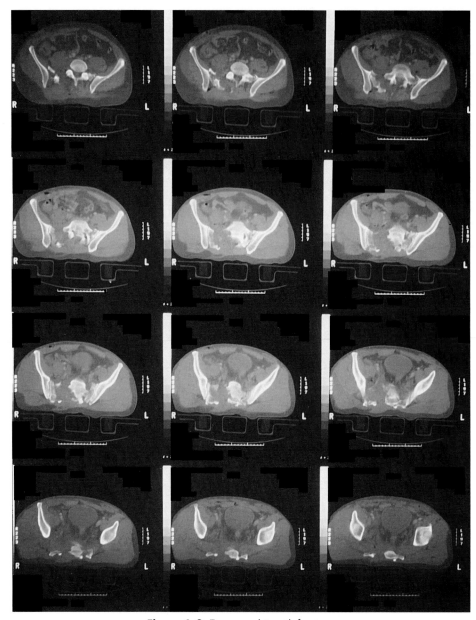

Figure 6–2. Trauma pelvis with fractures

Chart 6–3. **Musculoskeletal** (Fig. 6–3)

Pathology	Right iliac wing metastasizes from lung cancer
Description	Most common lesion of the bone; soft tissue lesion with erosion into the right iliac wing bone with a pathologic fracture present
Symptoms	History of cancer Pain in hip area
Suggested protocols	Routine pelvis to look at soft tissue component Reconstruction with bone algorithm to distinguish fracture
Appearance	Discontinuity of bone of iliac wing; soft tissue (gray) surrounding bone and displacing muscles and other structures
Contrast	To enhance lesion

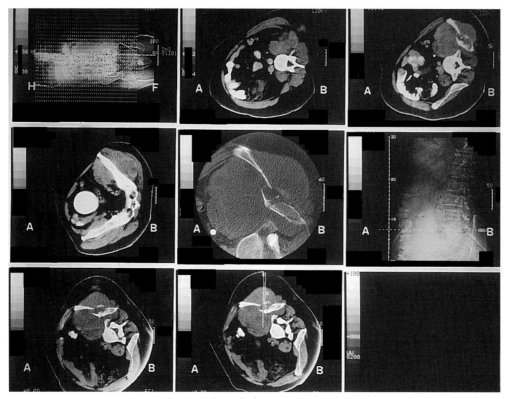

Figure 6-3. Right iliac wing metastases

Chart 6–4. **Musculoskeletal** (Figs. 6–4, 6–5)

Pathology	Right gluteal mass with invasion into iliac wing
Description	Differentials could be benign lesion of the skeletal muscle or an alveolar rhabdomyosarcoma (a highly malignant and rapidly growing lesion, usually found around shoulder and pelvis)
Symptoms	Palpable lesion, pain
Suggested protocols	Routine pelvis with larger than usual field of view
Appearance	Asymmetric gluteals with erosion into iliac wing
Contrast	To enhance lesion

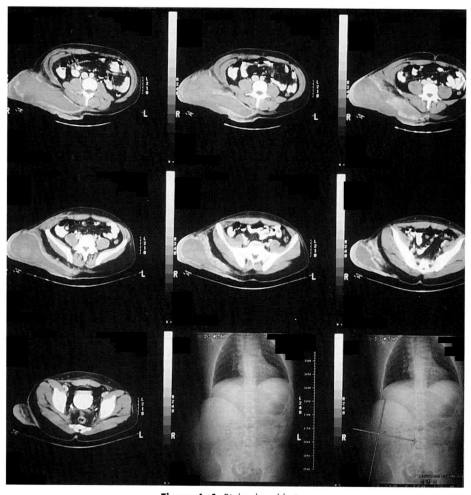

Figure 6–4. Right gluteal lesion

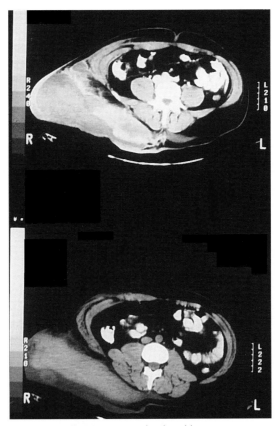

Figure 6–5. Right gluteal lesion

Chart 6–5. **Musculoskeletal** (Figs. 6–6, 6–7)

Pathology	Lytic lesion of tibia
Description	Characterized by destruction of red blood cells; differential diagnosis could be abscess, fibrous tumor, or metastasis
Symptoms	Leg pain
Suggested protocols	Routine extremity with 5-mm slices and small field of view
Appearance	Lesion appears dark in the grayish white bone
Contrast	To check for enhancement

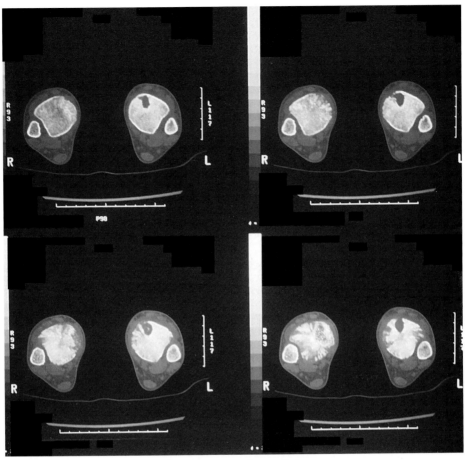

Figure 6–6. Lytic lesion of tibia

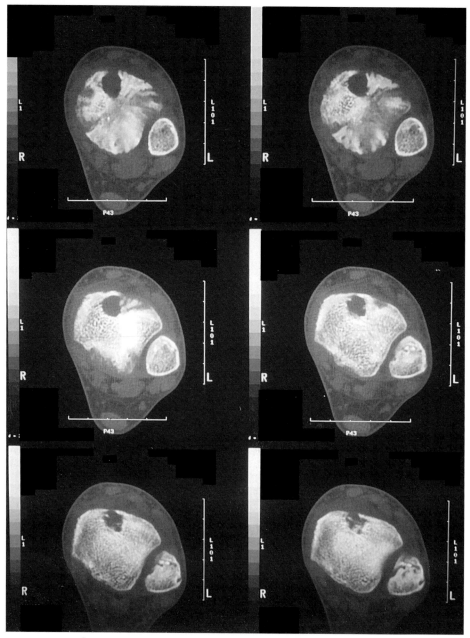

Figure 6–7. Lytic lesion of tibia

Chart 6–6. **Musculoskeletal** (Figs. 6–8 to 6–10)

Pathology	Severe distal tibia-fibula (ankle) fractures
Description	Trauma to ankle with displaced fractures of ankle (tibia and fibula)
Symptoms	Pain, swelling, trauma
Suggested protocols	mAs = 220 kVp = 120 Slice thickness = 4 mm Matrix = 256 × 256 DFOV = 160 mm
Appearance	Fracture lines are dark against grayish bone Bones are not in alignment
Contrast	Dependent on radiologist

mAs = milliampere-seconds; kVp = kilovolt (peak); DFOV = display field of view.

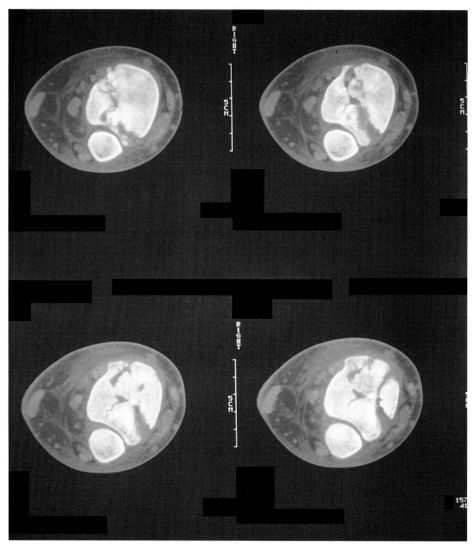

Figure 6-8. Ankle fracture

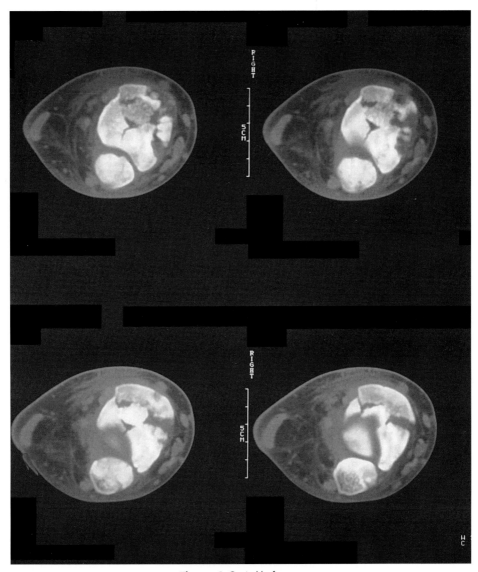

Figure 6–9. Ankle fracture

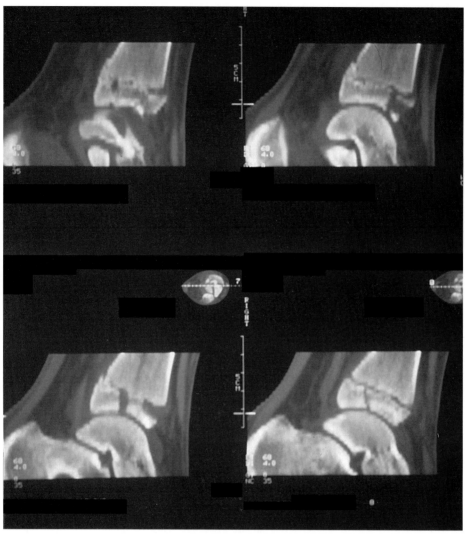

Figure 6–10. Sagittal reconstructions of ankle fractures

Chart 6–7. **Musculoskeletal** (Fig. 6–11)

Pathology	Calcaneus fracture
Description	Discontinuity of bone in calcaneus from trauma; CT performed to see placement of bone fragments
Symptoms	Trauma; swelling, unable to bear weight, pain
Suggested protocols	mAs = 210 kVp = 120 Matrix = 256 × 256 Slice thickness = 4 mm DFOV = 150 mm
Appearance	Fracture lines are dark in the grayish bone
Contrast	Dependent on radiologist

mAs = milliampere-seconds; kVp = kilovolt (peak); DFOV = display field of view.

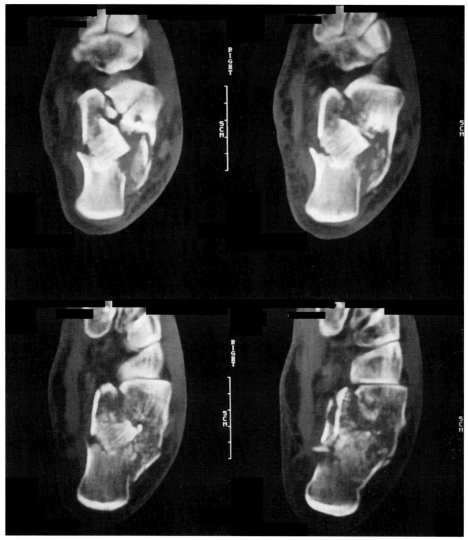

Figure 6–11. Calcaneus fracture

CHAPTER SEVEN

Summary

It is hoped that this pathology atlas enables you to delve into disease processes with more vigor. It has perhaps provided a solid background to research, study, and scan with additional tools the disease processes that interest you. I encourage each of you always to put yourself in your patients' shoes when coping with a serious disease process and the endless testing that comes with the diagnosis.

Index

Note: Page numbers in *italics* refer to illustrations.